Operation Crisis

OPERATION HEALTH

A SERIES OF BOOKS EXPLORING SURGERY AND GLOBAL HEALTH

Operation Crisis

Surgical Care in the Developing World

during Conflict and Disaster

EDITED BY

Adam L. Kushner, MD, MPH, FACS

JOHNS HOPKINS BLOOMBERG SCHOOL OF PUBLIC HEALTH

JOHNS HOPKINS UNIVERSITY PRESS   BALTIMORE

© 2017 Johns Hopkins University Press
All rights reserved. Published 2017
Printed in the United States of America on acid-free paper
9 8 7 6 5 4 3 2 1

Johns Hopkins University Press
2715 North Charles Street
Baltimore, Maryland 21218-4363
www.press.jhu.edu

Library of Congress Cataloging-in-Publication Data

Names: Kushner, Adam L., 1965– editor.
Title: Operation crisis : surgical care in the developing world during
    conflict and disaster / Adam L. Kushner, editor.
Other titles: Operation health (Series)
Description: Baltimore : Johns Hopkins University Press, 2017. | Series:
    Operation health | Includes bibliographical references and index.
Identifiers: LCCN 2016025745| ISBN 9781421422084 (pbk. : alk. paper) | ISBN
    9781421422091 (electronic) | ISBN 1421422085 (pbk. : alk. paper) | ISBN
    1421422093 (electronic)
Subjects: | MESH: Disaster Medicine—methods | Disasters | Armed Conflicts |
    Surgical Procedures, Operative | Developing Countries
Classification: LCC RD31.5 | NLM WA 295 | DDC 617.09172/4—dc23
    LC record available at https://lccn.loc.gov/2016025745

A catalog record for this book is available from the British Library.

*Special discounts are available for bulk purchases of this book. For more information, please
contact Special Sales at 410-516-6936 or specialsales@press.jhu.edu.*

Johns Hopkins University Press uses environmentally friendly book materials,
including recycled text paper that is composed of at least 30 percent post-consumer
waste, whenever possible.

Contents

Contributors

Kapendra Shekhar Amatya, MBBS, MS
Nepal Cancer Hospital and Research Center
Lalitpur, Nepal

Samer Attar, MD
Department of Orthopedics
Northwestern University
Chicago, IL, USA

Jeffrey A. Bailey, MD, FACS
COL, US Army
Joint Trauma System, Defense Center of Excellence
Fort Sam Houston, TX, USA
Department of Surgery
Uniformed Services University of the Health Sciences
Bethesda, MD, USA

Lucas C. Carlson, MD, MPH
Department of Emergency Medicine
Brigham & Women's Hospital
Boston, MA, USA

James C. Cobey, MD, MPH, FACS
Senior Associate
Johns Hopkins Bloomberg School of Public Health
Baltimore, MD, USA
Department of Orthopaedic Surgery
Georgetown University
Washington, DC, USA

Dattesh R. Dave, MD, MSc
Institute for Global Orthopaedics and Traumatology
San Francisco, CA, USA
Department of Orthopaedic Surgery
University of California, San Francisco, CA, USA

Dan L. Deckelbaum, MD, MPH, FACS
Co-director, Centre for Global Surgery
McGill University Health Centre
Montreal, Quebec, Canada

Richard A. Gosselin, MD, MPH, MSC, FRCS(C)
Institute for Global Orthopaedics and Traumatology
San Francisco, CA, USA
Department of Orthopaedic Surgery
University of California, San Francisco, CA, USA

Shailvi Gupta, MD, MPH
Department of Surgery
University of California, San Francisco–East Bay
Oakland, CA, USA
International Surgical Fellow
Surgeons OverSeas
New York, USA

Edna Adan Ismail, SRN, CMB, SCM
Founder and CEO
Edna Adan University Hospital
Chancellor, Edna Adan University
Hargeisa, Somaliland

Thaim B. Kamara, MBBS, FWACS
Department of Surgery
Connaught Hospital
Freetown, Sierra Leone

T. Peter Kingham, MD, FACS
Assistant Professor
Division of Hepatopancreatobiliary Surgery
Memorial Sloan Kettering Cancer Center
New York, NY, USA
President, Surgeons OverSeas
New York, NY, USA

Adam L. Kushner, MD, MPH, FACS
Founder and Director
Surgeons OverSeas
New York, NY, USA
Associate, Department of International Health
Johns Hopkins Bloomberg School of Public Health
Baltimore, MD, USA
Lecturer, Department of Surgery
Columbia University
New York, NY, USA

Judy M. Lee, MD, MPH, MBA, FACOG
Department of Gynecology and Obstetrics
Johns Hopkins Hospital
Baltimore, MD, USA

Maria "Tane" Pilar Luna, MD
Médecins Sans Frontières
Sydney, Australia

Brijesh Mishra, MS, MCh
King George's Medical University
Lucknow, Uttar Pradesh, India

Kyle N. Remick, MD, FACS
LTC, US Army
Trauma, Acute Care Surgery, Surgical Critical Care
Walter Reed National Military Medical Center
Uniformed Services University of the Health Sciences
Bethesda, MD, USA

Lauri J. Romanzi, MD, FACOG, FPMRS
Clinical Associate Professor
Department of Urology
NYU Langone Medical Center
New York, NY, USA

Michael Sinclair, MD, FACS
Médecins Sans Frontières / Doctors Without Borders—USA
New York, NY, USA

Barclay T. Stewart, MD, MscPH
Department of Surgery
University of Washington
Seattle, WA, USA

Marten van Wijhe, MD, PhD
Anesthesia advisor (retired)
Médecins Sans Frontières—OCA
Amsterdam, the Netherlands
Director Pain Management Unit (retired)
Department of Anesthesiology
University Hospital Groningen
Groningen, the Netherlands

Evan G. Wong, MD, MPH
Centre for Global Surgery
McGill University Health Centre
Montreal, Quebec, Canada
International Surgical Fellow
Surgeons OverSeas
New York, NY, USA

Series Editor's Foreword

I know someone who needed surgery. He was born by emergent cesarean section. He had urgent stomach surgery at 2 months and an appendectomy at 23.

He is alive today because of surgery. I am that person.

Throughout much of the world, the lack of surgical care leads to death or disability for millions of men, women, and children. Yet despite this reality, the global health community has not fully recognized the urgent need for improving surgical care. Surgery and anesthesia are integral to the treatment of traumatic injuries and obstructed labor. Many infectious complications need surgery. Surgery is often the best or only treatment for many cancers. During conflict and after disasters, populations are vulnerable and need surgical care. But millions of people around the world lack access to such care.

I cannot say exactly what led me to train as a surgeon and practice in the developing world. What I do know is that to prepare to practice overseas, in the middle of my surgical training, I obtained a master of public health degree from Johns Hopkins University. At that time—1998—there was almost no mention of surgery within public health. I remember knocking on dozens of doors. I asked everyone about public health research projects that included surgical care. Time after time no one could help me.

I was not discouraged. I felt there must be a need for surgical care and so finished my surgery training. For a decade I practiced and taught in countries ranging from Iraq to Indonesia, Sierra Leone to South Sudan, and Niger to Nicaragua. My public health training had included a great deal about infectious diseases such as HIV, tuberculosis, and malaria. The reality that I began to see was that surgical care was also needed. I treated women in obstructed labor, children with appendicitis and typhoid perforations, and adults with fractures, hernias, and cancer. Many of these patients presented with late-stage disease. I began to wonder, How many patients were not seeking care? How many were dying in their villages and fields? How many were not as fortunate as I?

In 2008, along with local colleagues, I began documenting deficiencies in providing surgical care. A study in Sierra Leone showed no compressed oxygen, limited quantities of sterile gloves and eye protection, and only 10 surgeons for a population of 6 million. We showed that Sierra Leone hospitals in 2008 were worse off than US Civil War hospitals in 1864. Later, we conducted population-based surveys of surgical need in Sierra Leone, Rwanda, and Nepal. Estimates showed that up to 25% of the populations needed an operation and that access to surgery might have averted up to 33% of deaths. We had begun providing the evidence showing that millions of people around the world needed and wanted surgical care.

In 2013, I began teaching a course called "Surgical Care Needs in Low and Middle Income Countries" at the Johns Hopkins Bloomberg School of Public Health. The course covered surgical epidemiology, surgery for women and children, and surgical care during conflict and disasters. It was one of the first global surgery courses taught in the United States and the first at Johns Hopkins. Surgery and anesthesia had finally made a toehold in public health.

The course also led to Johns Hopkins University Press publishing *Operation Health: Surgical Care in the Developing World*. It was the first book in what would become the Operation Health series. The chapters begin with a personal vignette; then, experts from around the globe present case studies, best practices, and topic overviews. Chapters cover subjects such as cesarean sections in Ethiopia, clubfoot in Nepal, trauma in Tanzania, anesthesia in Ghana, and laparoscopy in Mongolia. The book is meant to speak to clinicians, students, and the general public. I hoped that it would educate and enlighten readers who would care about global surgery, many of whom just didn't yet know they cared.

With the success and interest generated by the first book, I developed a series covering the various aspects of the massive surgical needs in the developing world. Future books will cover conflict and disasters; cancer; women's health; child health; surgical subspecialties; anesthesia and critical care; and even surgical care and Ebola. Following the blueprint of the first book, each volume will be short, suitable for students, clinicians, and the interested general public.

As the field of global surgery matures within global health, the question is not *should* we provide surgical care but *how*. By providing rich and accessible overviews alongside lessons learned from personal experiences, the Operation Health series begins to provide some ways forward.

Adam L. Kushner, MD, MPH, FACS

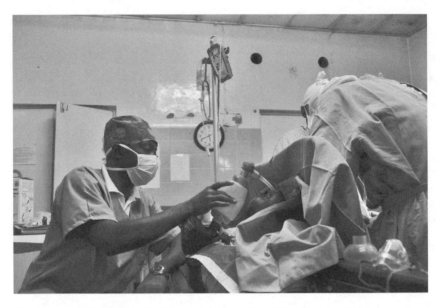

P.1. An operation in the Democratic Republic of the Congo. Photo courtesy Chiels Liu

Preface

Hippocrates advised, "He who wishes to be a surgeon should go to war." No clinical setting requires such a combination of good surgical skills, teamwork, and poise under pressure as during war. To ably care for patients using limited resources in a disrupted health system, healthcare personnel must develop special abilities and use techniques that differ from "normal" conditions.

Historically, many important advances in wound care and injury management were developed and improved during times of conflict. Ambroise Paré, a French barber-surgeon in the mid-1500s, was one of the first to repair injured blood vessels and to bandage wounds instead of using cauterization. Though the advances were beneficial, he also noted, "I bandaged them, but god healed them."

Other advances during wartime included the development of rapid evacuation, trauma systems, damage control resuscitation, and damage control surgery. Using these advances in Iraq and Afghanistan, the US military has reduced the battlefield mortality rate to less than 5%, a historic low. These advances, technologies, resources, and transport systems, however, are not available to the majority of civilian victims in the developing world.

Although the media often portray the heroic efforts of international surgical teams that travel to conflict and disaster zones, it is important to recognize that local healthcare workers provide the majority of care. International medical personnel working for organizations such as the International Committee of the Red Cross (ICRC) and Médecins Sans Frontières (MSF, also known as Doctors Without Borders) arrive later. These volunteers must be able to adapt to the local context and, most importantly, practice the medical dictum of *primum non nocere*: "First, do no harm."

Surgical care is increasingly recognized as an important part of global health, but few surgeons are involved in global health efforts. It is essential to inform public health professionals, provide useful descriptions of the context, and define issues that surround global surgical care. As part of the Johns Hopkins University Press Operation Health series, the present volume focuses on providing surgical care in war zones and after disasters. The book is divided into three sections: Personal Perspectives, Surgical Care Principles, and A Way Forward.

Part I provides personal insights and overviews of the context. Chapter 1 is by a local surgeon who cared for injured victims of the 2015 Nepal earthquake. Subsequent chapters are by an international orthopedic surgeon, general surgeons, and an obstetrician-gynecologist. Chapters 3 and 4 are accounts based on MSF missions. For more than 40 years, MSF has sent volunteers to war and disaster zones, and many students dream of working with them. These chapters highlight the needs and limitations, but also detail the type of work that can be accomplished.

Part II covers various surgical care principles required for providing care during crisis, including triage and training, wounds and fractures, burn care, anesthesia, women's health, and sexual violence.

Part III looks at ways to move forward. Chapter 11 provides an overview of how the data collection for land mine injuries helped establish the Mine Ban Treaty. Chapter 12 focuses on lessons learned in the aftermath of the Haiti earthquake. Chapter 13 covers the US military Joint Trauma System and shows what can be accomplished with increased resources and the political will to provide care. The high quality of care that US battlefield casualties receive is in stark contrast to what most civilians receive during a crisis.

As in other books in the Operation Health series, experienced healthcare personnel wrote the chapters. The stories are personal and frequently disturbing, but that is the nature of conflict and the aftermath of a disaster. In high-income countries, surgical care is thought of as excessively expensive and complicated; however, this does not have to be the case. Simple, safe, and appropriate care can be and is provided in developing countries during conflict and after disasters. To better understand the context and to understand how to plan and prepare, a public health approach is useful. In this book, chapters roughly follow the format of a personal story or experience and then a more detailed description of the magnitude of the problem. Possible interventions help to offer solutions and ways to improve care for future victims of crisis.

The goal of this book is to highlight the provision of surgical care during conflict and disaster for public health, medical, and nursing students interested in studying the topic and for the general reader who wants to know more about the context. By no means is this book a formal "how to" manual. Other works describing the technical aspects already exist. This book is intended to spark further discussion and highlight situations where surgical care can save lives and reduce disability. It also provides insights into the role of surgical health care, functions as an advocacy tool, and provides recommendations for a way forward.

Increased awareness can lead to greater surgical care resources for personnel, equipment, supplies, and training, which will save lives and reduce disabilities. It is hoped that this book helps in that effort.

Operation Crisis

I   PERSONAL PERSPECTIVES

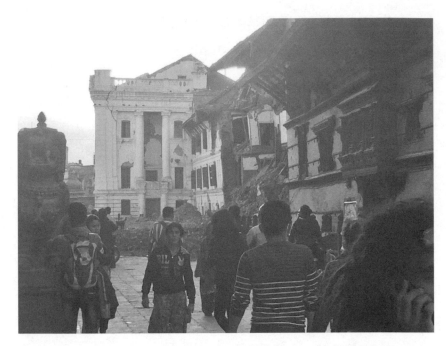

1.1. Destruction of the UNESCO World Heritage site Basantapur Palace Square after the 2015 Nepal earthquake. Photo courtesy Kapendra Shekhar Amatya

1

Surgical Care after the April 2015 Nepal Earthquake

KAPENDRA SHEKHAR AMATYA, MBBS, MS

I work as a surgeon at a cancer hospital in Nepal. On April 25, 2015, at 11:56 a.m., a 7.8-magnitude earthquake struck. In the immediate aftermath, my main job was to discharge patients who could be managed at home and provide shelter to the patients still needing care. Shortly afterward we had an influx of trauma patients from a severely damaged village nearby. Without an adequate operating room, we could only provide basic wound care, X-rays, minor debridements, and dressing on an outpatient basis. The severely wounded patients were referred to the functioning tertiary centers nearby.

Safeguarding cancer patients already present at the hospital continued to be our main function, but we quickly built makeshift hospitals. By the end of the first week, organized teams were providing health services to the affected areas of Lalitpur District. Our aim was to treat wounds and distribute medicines to people who could not afford such care or who were unable to travel to a hospital.

It took three months for our hospital to return to normal.

The earthquake, with an epicenter east of Lamjung District, was at a shallow depth of 8.2 km (5.1 mi). It was the worst natural disaster to strike the region since the Nepal-Bihar earthquake in 1934. The April earthquake triggered a huge avalanche in the Langtang Valley, where 250 people went missing. Hundreds of thousands of people were left homeless, with entire villages flattened. Centuries-old buildings were destroyed at UNESCO World Heritage sites in the Kathmandu Valley, including the Kathmandu Durbar Square, the Patan Durbar Square, the Bhaktapur Durbar Square, the Changu

Narayan Temple, and the Swayambhunath Stupa. In addition, an avalanche on Mount Everest killed at least 19, making it the deadliest single day on the mountain in history.

Continued aftershocks occurred at intervals of 15 to 20 minutes. One aftershock on April 26 reached a magnitude of 6.7. Another major aftershock of 7.3 occurred on May 12. In total, more than 8,800 persons died and nearly three times as many were injured.

Although Nepal had been warned about the possibility of this kind of earthquake, many people refused to believe it would happen and many were unprepared. This was also true for the medical community. Many hospitals were ill prepared and underequipped to handle the crisis. The aftermath of the earthquake unfolded into three periods: acute, subacute, and chronic.

Acute

The earthquake shook Nepal on Saturday, the official holiday of the week. At all hospitals this means limited in-house physicians and staff. Yet despite this being a day off, most physicians, nurses, and support personnel reported to their respective facilities within a few hours of the disaster.

What they saw on arrival at the hospitals was something each would never forget. The main hospitals in the Kathmandu Valley were flooded with victims. Some of the hospital buildings were also damaged, so patients needed to be referred or transferred to functioning facilities with stable structures. No special triage systems were in place, and very few staff knew how to handle mass casualty situations. While initial accounts from various hospitals differed in specific details, the majority gave a similar overall picture.

In the first few hours after the earthquake, the medical teams were mainly focused on distinguishing between people who were dead or alive. As the aftershocks were still ongoing, only very dire emergency operations were carried out. Most of the initial interventions were limited to primary and basic trauma care. This included stabilization, resuscitation, basic wound management and dressings, debridements, and plaster fixation for fractures. The limited stock of medicines and supplies caused havoc in the hospitals. Theft of supplies and medication from hospital pharmacies and storerooms was also reported.

Fortunately, the Nepal government announced free medical care for all persons injured by the earthquake. Patients, clinicians, and hospital administrators were all greatly relieved by this policy, which allowed many to be treated. Within days, makeshift wards and operating rooms were established in tents on hospital grounds and more sophisticated treatments were started. These included internal repair of fractures, complex debridements, fixation of spinal injuries, and amputations. Most of the hospitals had stopped all their regular elective surgeries to focus on earthquake-related trauma services. Hospitals also developed mobile health teams to provide services to areas most affected by the earthquake.

By the end of the first week, international medical teams began arriving and providing humanitarian medical care. Some international volunteers performed surgical operations, but more importantly they brought fresh stocks of medications and medical supplies.

Subacute

By the second and into the third week, most of the victims had received primary trauma care. Within this time period the powerful 7.3 aftershock shook Nepal again. This aggravated the fear among both the people and the medical personnel. This time it was on a working day, and most of the surgeons were operating when the earth shook. Despite the danger, the medical relief carried on.

At this time, the operations were more and more complex and included internal fixation of fractures, debridements, fixation of spinal injuries, and amputations that had been delayed. Another significant part of the surgical workload was treatment of victims brought from remote areas of the country who had had a difficult time accessing the main cities. Most of these patients had received primary care in their primary healthcare centers, but they now needed tertiary care. Hospitals continued to provide health services in the affected areas via outreach, mobile clinics, and medical camps. Most of the hospitals also slowly restarted their regular services.

By the third week the community service at our hospital was functioning well and the hospital team under my supervision was able to provide continuous health care to six village development centers with the collaboration of primary health centers in the region.

I remember a shelter where elderly patients received care. We continuously provided wound care for four weeks until the patients were able to take care of themselves. One 83-year-old woman with an intertrochanteric fracture of her right femur refused to go to a hospital. A makeshift bed and traction were fashioned in the shelter with materials available at the site. Unfortunately, she passed away after the third week due to her deteriorating condition.

Once the immediate medical needs of the patients were dealt with, we began to recognize the importance of providing clean drinking water and proper sanitation. Within five weeks our medical team in cooperation with the Rotary Club and other donor agencies was able to provide facilities for both. We also provided materials for personal hygiene such as soap, toothpaste and toothbrushes, and sanitary pads. This greatly helped stop any infectious diseases that we were afraid might develop.

Chronic

Nearly one and half months after the earthquake, many hospitals were able to return to relatively regular work routines. They were still busy with victims of the disaster, but the types of operations changed to focusing on rehabilitation and improving the functional outcome after traumatic injury. Cases included internal fixation removals and skin grafting of large wounds. These types of cases and rehabilitation services were still carried out up to six months after the earthquake. It will take a long time to fully recover from all the trauma of the devastation, and a scar will remain in the heart of all the people of Nepal for a long time to come.

Additional insights for this chapter were provided by the personal experience of Dr. Nabees Man Singh Pradhan, Consultant Orthopedic Surgeon, Patan Hospital, Lalitpur, Nepal, and Dr. Romeo Kansakar, Janamaitri Hospital, Kathmandu, Nepal.

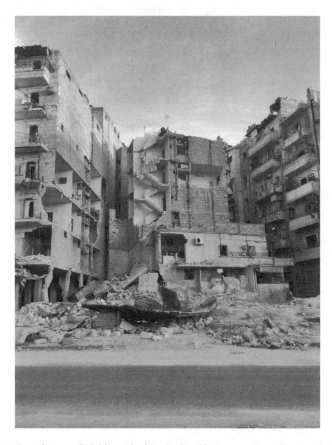

2.1. View from a field hospital in Syria. Photo courtesy Samer Attar

2

A Health System Destroyed

Surgical Care in Syria

SAMER ATTAR, MD, AND SHAILVI GUPTA, MD, MPH

An oil drum filled with nails, stones, and explosives—a barrel bomb—was pushed from a helicopter onto the house where a father and son slept. This inexpensive yet devastating weapon destroyed their home. Neighbors and volunteers rushed to the scene to search for survivors. Both the father and the son survived the blast. They were carried down rubble-strewn streets under the threat of snipers to a makeshift hospital in Aleppo, Syria.

Both father and son required bilateral above-the-knee amputations. Four limbs—two lives forever shattered. After beginning to heal, the boy asked for new legs. Despite the surrounding destruction, he thought prosthetic limbs were delivered like shoes. He thought, or maybe hoped, his life would return to normal. Unfortunately, during conflict, health systems are severely disrupted and most victims requiring surgical care do not get adequate treatment or the rehabilitation they need.

Since March 2011, a civil war has consumed Syria. Over 10 million people have been displaced from their homes, with over 3 million refugees in Turkey, Jordan, and Lebanon. At the start of 2015, the death toll exceeded 200,000 persons, with an additional 1 million injured. Before the conflict, the most common cause of death was similar to other middle- and high-income countries—cardiovascular disease. Now gunshot wounds, artillery shells, and barrel bombs top the list. Throughout Syria, in cities like Aleppo, snipers perch on rooftops and target the vulnerable: children and the elderly. Children are shot in the head while walking with their parents; others are shot in the abdomen. A report by Johns Hopkins University researchers documented a 50% decrease in clinic visits and surgical cases; injured civilians often forgo needed care due to risks from snipers and bombs, and from fear of security forces who arrest the wounded in public hospitals.

In addition to the targeting of civilians, more than 600 medical personnel deaths were reported from bombings, sniper fire, execution, or torture. Healthcare workers have also fled the country. As of early 2015, only 100 physicians remained in Aleppo, a city that previously had 2,500. The resulting shortage of physicians, particularly surgeons, is reflected in the large number of deaths and especially an increase in the number of amputations. With more sophisticated care and better-trained personnel, many lives and limbs could be saved.

Although protected by international humanitarian law, hospitals and health facilities are targeted. The bombings destroy critical healthcare infrastructure and equipment, and they inhibit resupply and repair. As of August 2014, only 45% of Syria's public hospitals were fully operational, 34% were functioning partially, and 21% were not functioning at all.

An ideal healthcare system delivers quality services to all people when and where there is a need. Prevention, immediate care, and posttreatment opportunities, including rehabilitation and secondary prevention, are available. In Syria this is not the case. By September 2014 most pharmacies had closed, dialysis centers were open only a few days a week, and anesthesia and chronic disease medications were scarce.

Because of the assault on the healthcare system, makeshift health facilities were set up in apartment buildings, farms, and even caves. Although these makeshift facilities were called "field hospitals," many lacked the necessary medical and surgical equipment and expertise to adequately treat the large volume of casualties. These facilities, located close to the front lines, were staffed by a handful of doctors and surgeons, and volunteers without formal training. Few field hospitals had basic X-ray equipment; almost none had a CT scanner. Though a limited number of field hospitals have become relatively sophisticated over time with equipment provided by humanitarian organizations, such facilities cannot replace a well-established healthcare system. For most facilities, essential items such as intensive care units, ultrasound machines, and even oxygen and electricity are absent. Despite these limitations, field hospitals have been vital to the care of war wounded in Syria.

Life in a Syrian field hospital was exhausting, unforgiving, and at times horrifying. An unending stream of patients with mangled limbs, exposed organs, and crushed skulls arrived daily. Equipment and supplies were scarce. Complex care and rehabilitation were nonexistent. The care was vastly different from what is normally provided in high-income countries. The sounds of gunfire rarely stopped, and nearby blasts frequently shook a building's foundations. Occasionally, missiles and mortars landed on the doorstep. Wounded patients were placed two to a bed—side by side. When all beds were full, new arrivals were placed on the bloodstained floor. With insufficient operating rooms, surgeons operated on patients lying on stretchers in hallways. When the power went out, cell phones and portable headlamps provided light. Staff lived in the hospital, slept on the floor, and rarely changed out of scrubs.

The numbers of war wounded requiring surgical care quickly overwhelms these facilities. In Aleppo in early 2014, one field hospital averaged 50 to 75 war-related cases per day. One surgeon reportedly performed 11 amputations, mostly on children, in a single day. Like most victims of conflict, patients in Syria often arrive at field hospitals having received limited first aid. Since all war wounds are considered contaminated, they cannot be quickly closed. Delayed closure, after initial cleaning and debridement, is the norm. Frequently, these patients also lose a great deal of blood and may be in shock. Long operations are unwise. Adequate resuscitation with quick, temporizing, life- and limb-saving surgery is key. In addition, the possibility of additional victims and the lack of resources rarely allow for long definitive treatments or protracted and complex operations. If there is the possibility of stabilization and transfer to other facilities with better resources and staff, this is highly recommended. Unfortunately, for most civilians in Syria, onward transport is rarely an option.

When caring for victims of conflict, healthcare workers ideally have sufficient skills and knowledge before the onset of hostilities. Proper training in the management of war wounds and working with limited resources is essential, though frequently lacking among volunteers or inexperienced clinicians. Programs to prepare for such situations should be implemented along with the stockpiling of materials whenever disaster management personnel plan for mass casualty incidents. Courses on the care of war wounded should cover wound debridement, splinting, amputations, and external fixation of long bones. Skills and knowledge of other co-morbidities (e.g., diabetes) are also important during conflict. If the general health of patients cannot be maintained, simply providing surgical care may be a futile endeavor.

Providing quality surgical care always requires a team and systems approach; this extends throughout the conflict. Surgeons by themselves are capable of little. To adequately and safely care for wounded patients, there needs to be good preoperative evaluation and resuscitation, adequate and safe anesthesia, skilled nursing, and proper wound care.

Prehospital care, first aid, and long-term rehabilitation all help to improve the chances that a victim will recover and be successfully reintegrated into society. During active combat all these conditions are difficult to achieve. But if a limited system is established, then a better recovery is more likely after the cessation of hostilities or in the reconstruction phase after a disaster.

In planning for postconflict Syria, resources and focus will be crucial to redevelop the healthcare system. With the current disruption of care, local leaders, clinicians, and the international community must take reconstruction into account before the end of the conflict. In the long term, stronger health systems improve the health of the population, in turn leading to greater productivity and economic growth, less violence, and state stability—all necessary components for successful postconflict rebuilding of Syria.

Oftentimes, health interventions during conflict rely on humanitarian relief, which provides immediate assistance but does not necessarily advance health system development; donors have not necessarily made health system development a priority, as humanitarian relief often appears more urgent and vital than long-term health system rebuilding, and investments in states are fragile. Despite the difficulties and limitations, efforts to strengthen health systems during conflict are essential. Efforts must be made to train frontline health workers, provide adequate resources, and provide long-term rehabilitation. Without such effort, children with amputated limbs will not receive the prosthetics they need and injured parents will be unable to provide for their families.

Samer Attar, MD, is an orthopedic surgeon at Northwestern Hospital in Chicago, IL. In August 2013 and April 2014, he volunteered with the Syrian American Medical Society and worked in the "m10" field hospital in Aleppo, Syria.

ADDITIONAL READING

Alahdab F, Omar MH, Alsakka S, Al-Moujahed A, Atassi B. Syrians' alternative to health care system: "field hospitals." *Avicenna Journal of Medicine*, 4, no. 3 (2014): 51–52.

Barriga SR. Dispatches: invisible victims of the Syrian conflict—people with disabilities. Human Rights Watch. September 19, 2013. *http://www.hrw.org /news/2013/09/19/dispatches-invisible-victims-syrian-conflict-people-disabilities* (accessed March 5, 2016).

Brundtland GH, Glinka E, zur Hausen H, d'Avila RL. Open letter: let us treat patients in Syria. *Lancet* (2013) 382: 1019–1020.

Coupland RM. *War wounds of limbs: surgical management.* International Committee of the Red Cross, Geneva, Switzerland, 1993.

Giannou C, Bladan M. *War surgery: working with limited resources in armed conflict and other situations of violence*, vol. 1. International Committee of the Red Cross, Geneva, Switzerland, 2009.

Giannou C, Bladan M, Molde A. *War Surgery: working with limited resources in armed conflict and other situations of violence*, vol.2. International Committee of the Red Cross, Geneva, Switzerland, 2013.

Gray R. *War wounds: basic surgical management: principles and practice of the surgical management of wounds produced by missiles or explosions.* International Committee of the Red Cross, Geneva, Switzerland, 1994.

Haar RJ, Rubenstein LS. *Health in postconflict and fragile states.* United States Institute of Peace, Special Report. January 2012.

Kherallah M, Alahfez T, Sahloul Z, Eddin KD, Jamil G. Syrian International Coalition for Health, Global Health Equity Foundation, Geneva. *Avicenna Journal of Medicine* 2, no. 3 (2012).

Salama H, Dardagan H. *Stolen futures: the hidden toll of child casualties in Syria.* Oxford Research Group. November 24, 2014. *http://www.oxfordresearchgroup.org.uk/ publications/briefing_papers_and_reports/stolen_futures* (accessed March 5, 2016).

Syrian medical voices from the ground: the ordeal of Syria's healthcare professionals. Center for Public Health and Human Rights, Johns Hopkins Bloomberg School of Public Health, Syrian American Medical Society, February 2015.

United National Human Rights Council. *Assault on medical care in Syria* (A/HRC/24/ CRP.2). ReliefWeb. September 13, 2013. *http://reliefweb.int/report/syrian-arab -republic/assault-medical-care-syria-ahrc24crp2* (accessed March 5, 2016).

World Health Organization. *Donor update: Syrian Arab Republic.* September 2013, Quarter 3 Report. *http://www.who.int/hac/syria_donorupdate_18102013.pdf* (accessed March 5, 2016).

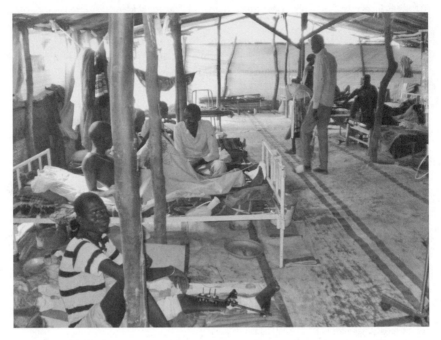

3.1. Surgical ward, Doctors Without Borders / Médecins Sans Frontières Hospital, Lankien, South Sudan. Photo courtesy Michael Sinclair

3

A Surgeon's Day in South Sudan

MICHAEL SINCLAIR, MD, FACS

It was a few minutes before 8 a.m., and I quickly made rounds through the crowded tent that functioned as the surgical ward. After a hurried breakfast and the morning meeting with expatriate and national staff, I was only able to spend a few moments seeing patients before rushing to the operating room. This was a Doctors Without Borders / Médecins Sans Frontières (MSF) hospital managed by Operational Center Amsterdam in Lankien, South Sudan. I was the only surgeon. On the ward, I could only "put out fires."

With an average daily census of 120 to 130 surgical patients, I only saw the sickest patients, the ones who had had a recent operation, or who the nurses asked me to review. I had little help—there were no residents, clinical officers, or other ancillary personnel.

After rounds and once in the operating room, porters brought several patients to an anteroom that functioned as a preoperative evaluation area. The space was merely a tent connected to the inflatable structure that was the operating and recovery rooms. Neither the pre-op area nor recovery room had beds, suction, or resuscitative equipment or supplies.

The day's operative schedule included:

1. Child with 20% body surface area burns for debridement and dressing change
2. Child with snakebite of the hand for debridement, partial wound closure, and dressing change
3. Adult male for skin graft of arm and leg wounds (after multiple debridements, his wounds were now clean)

4. Adult male with a large tissue defect over an exposed fracture of the tibia and fibula for a muscle flap and skin graft
5. Adult male for debridement plus external fixation of an open fracture of the humerus
6. Adult male for debridement of osteomyelitis (bone infection) of the femur
7   Adult male needing an operation for an incarcerated inguinal hernia
8. Adult male for incision and drainage of a severe hand infection

If there were no emergencies, the team would break for lunch at noon and the scheduled cases would finish by 5 or 6 p.m., but that was unlikely. Nearly every day, the scheduled cases were delayed because of new emergency cases. These new cases could be patients with acute appendicitis or more commonly, gunshot wounds.

South Sudan became the world's newest nation and formally gained independence from Sudan in July 2011. After a two-decade-long civil war that devastated infrastructure, healthcare, education, and development, hopes were high that conditions would improve. Obstacles to progress were formidable, but many governments and nongovernmental organizations (NGOs) offered funding and technical assistance. A fledgling Ministry of Health was responsible for the health system, but much of the healthcare was provided or heavily supported by international NGOs. For surgical care, MSF and the International Committee of the Red Cross (ICRC) were the most prominent organizations.

In December 2013, long-standing ethnic and tribal rivalries erupted into an armed conflict between forces loyal to the government and those supporting an ousted vice president. Fighting began in the capital, Juba, and rapidly spread to the surrounding states. The violence compounded problems with the already fragile and overburdened healthcare system. As fighting intensified, even health facilities were targeted and destroyed.

With the outbreak of hostilities, MSF, which already had a substantial presence in the country, responded by increasing the number of expatriate and national staff and changing the focus of programs to meet the increase in war-wounded patients. For 25 years, MSF ran a hospital in the village of Leer. In January 2014, the village, including the hospital, was looted and burned. MSF staff were forced to flee into the bush, taking patients with them and caring for them for several weeks while in hiding. Later, a Ministry of Health–run hospital in Malakal was abandoned when antigovernment forces overran the city. After the Ministry of Health personnel fled, another MSF team entered the city and provided medical and surgical services on the hospital grounds. Increased violence forced the team to move to an adjacent United Nations compound, where a makeshift hospital and refugee camp were established.

With the spreading violence, movement of personnel and supplies, normally complicated by a poor transportation infrastructure, became worse. Small aircraft that could land on dirt airstrips in remote locations became the only source of resupply. Despite these logistical limitations, in January 2014, MSF leadership sought to establish a new surgical program in the village of Lankien, the site of a long-standing medical, pediatric, nutrition, and antenatal/obstetrical project. This hospital would become the only facility providing surgical care for hundreds of thousands of patients in northern Jonglei State, South Sudan.

Initially, there was no space for surgical patients or for an operating room, because the hospital was already full with medical patients. As few building materials were available, surgical wards were hastily constructed using tents. Nonsurgical patients were crowded together to make room for the influx of wounded patients requiring surgical care. At first, the majority of the surgical patients lay on blankets on the ground, because there were an insufficient number of beds. A specialized inflatable tent arrived and was used as an operating room. In late January, a surgeon, anesthesiologist, and operating room nurse arrived in Lankien and the surgical program began.

As is typical in rural African hospitals and temporary facilities during conflict, the hospital had no X-ray, ultrasound machine, or blood bank. The only laboratory tests available were hemoglobin determination, checking blood group, and screening blood for HIV, hepatitis, syphilis, and malaria. There were no ventilators and no monitors except for digital pulse oximetry. There was no intensive care unit. There was no electrocautery in the operating room and only a single foot-pump-operated suction machine, shared by both the surgeon and anesthesiologist. Inhalational anesthesia was not available. All surgical procedures including amputations, cesarean sections, and abdominal operations were performed under local, spinal, or ketamine anesthesia. (For more detailed discussion on women's health, see Chapters 4 and 9, and for anesthesia, see Chapter 8.)

By the time I arrived in Lankien in early April, the surgical wards were overflowing and an average of eight operations were performed daily. In addition to the heavy workload, patient care was challenging, because the South Sudanese staff working on the wards and in the operating room were inexperienced. Shortages existed for basic equipment such as adhesive tape, bandages, exam gloves, and sterile gloves, as well as specialized surgical equipment to treat patients with complex fractures. The medical, pediatric, and obstetric-gynecological wards also suffered from insufficient supplies.

Approximately three-quarters of the surgical patients treated in Lankien were victims of war wounds—mostly from high-velocity gunshot wounds (AK-47) or shrapnel from rocket-propelled grenades (RPGs). The vast majority of surgical patients were young men, but I also treated two 8-year-old children and three women: two young and one elderly. Extremity wounds were the most common injury, usually open fractures from gunshot wounds. These fractures in this context were always contaminated and required multiple debridements and, if available, external fixation (an erector set–like device to stabilize broken bones until healing). Most femur (thigh) fractures were treated with skeletal traction, which requires two months of bed rest for proper healing. In a few instances external fixation was used for femur fractures as well. Internal fixation was not available and would not have been appropriate, because these wounds were grossly contaminated and operating room hygiene was not adequate for insertion of surgical hardware or other devices. Several lower-extremity fractures had exposed bone that required tissue flaps for coverage. Skin grafts were needed for many patients, and these operations were all performed with a handheld dermatome (Humby knife) since there were no electric devices. (For more detailed discussions on wounds and fractures, see Chapter 6.)

The patients were "self-triaged" in the sense that long delays in transfer to the hospital (days to even weeks) were the rule. I saw no patients with significant vascular injury, war-related head injuries, or major chest trauma; they most likely died before reaching the hospital. One young man was admitted with paraplegia from a gunshot wound. Two patients required laparotomies for neglected penetrating abdominal gunshot wounds. Both had extensive intra-abdominal sepsis, which led to prolonged, difficult postoperative courses. Fortunately, both survived. (For more details on triage, see Chapter 5.)

The non-conflict-related conditions requiring surgical care included snakebites, spider bites, burns, incarcerated hernias, soft tissue infections, appendicitis, and acute abdominal emergencies. There were also numerous obstetrical emergencies.

Only the simplest dressing changes were performed on the surgical ward because of difficulty in maintaining hygiene. Most patients were brought to the operating rooms, where they received heavy sedation or a brief general anesthetic while the wounds were evaluated, perhaps briefly debrided, and the dressings changed.

On Sunday the team had a "day off," performing only life-saving operations. An attempt was made to avoid operating at night if possible.

Because of the practical impossibility of reaching Lankien by ground transport (except for a small number of patients who could walk to the hospital from the nearby villages), most patients were transferred from remote "outreach" clinics by MSF aircraft. Often that referral system resulted in 6 to 16 surgical admissions on a single day. The periodic influx of war-wounded patients created havoc with the operating schedule. There was no "elective" surgery. Most trauma patients, especially those with burns, required multiple operations. The operating schedule was frequently full with planned "returns" for debridements, dressing changes, and other necessary, but not emergency, cases.

Providing surgical care in rural South Sudan was always difficult, and more so during active conflict. Deficiencies in supplies, equipment, and experienced personnel made providing safe surgical care problematic. Security for the team was also a major consideration, as fighting could affect the facility at any time. Though there was an evacuation plan for international staff, the community would certainly suffer if the staff left. Yet despite all the limitations, the project in Lankien proved that a small, dedicated surgical team supported by compassionate administrative and logistical colleagues can provide life- and limb-saving surgery for conflict victims and the population at large. Apart from following set protocols and knowing the principles of war surgery, successful surgical programs in a challenging environment, such as in rural South Sudan during conflict, require the ability to adapt, prioritize, and compromise.

Michael Sinclair, MD, FACS, is a retired cardiothoracic surgeon with extensive experience working in conflict and postconflict settings. He spent six weeks at the Médecins Sans Frontières hospital in Lankien, South Sudan, in April and May 2014.

ADDITIONAL READING

Anesthesia in resource-poor settings: the Médecins Sans Frontières experience. *The role of anesthesiology in global health.* Roth R, Frost EAM, Gevirtz C, *Atcheson CLH*, 2014. http://link.springer.com/chapter/10.1007%2F978-3-319-09423-6_9.

Surgery for victims of war, 3rd ed., Dufour D, Jensen S Kromann, Salmela J, Stening GF, Zetterstrom B, Molde A. International Committee of the Red Cross, Geneva, Switzerland, 1998.

War surgery in Afghanistan and Iraq: a series of cases, 2003–2007 (Textbooks of Military Medicine). Shawn Christian Nessen, MD (Editor), Stephen P. Hetz, MD (Editor), Bob Woodruff (Foreword). Walter Reed Army Medical Center Bordon Institute, 2008.

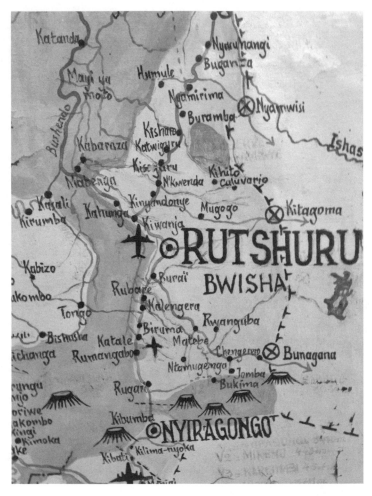

4.1. Map of Rutshuru, Democratic Republic of the Congo. Photo courtesy Maria "Tane" Pilar Luna

4

An Obstetrician in the Field

Some Lessons Learned

MARIA "TANE" PILAR LUNA, MD

Lesson 1: Welcome to Reality

She was 14 when she arrived with her mother at Benson Hospital in Monrovia, Liberia. It was November 2008, during my first mission with Médecins Sans Frontières (MSF). She presented with severe abdominal pain and fever. The mother told me that her daughter was pregnant and had gone to a local healer for procedures to terminate the pregnancy. After an initial assessment, I determined that she had a severe abdominal infection and needed surgery. The infection was probably secondary to the termination procedure.

We took her to the operating room (OR). At that point, the most important decision was whether the level of infection in her uterus required its removal or not. The infection seemed to be localized, so I decided on damage control, removing only the infected tissues and waiting for the antibiotics to complete the task of fighting the infection.

A few days later we were again in the OR; the infection was not getting any better and the uterus was still badly infected, so I had to remove it. Two more surgeries were needed in the following days for different complications. The girl's condition worsened every day, and we were all wondering what else could be done within our own capacities and limits. I will always remember that after the final operation I told her mother to go and get some rest. She thanked me but said that she preferred to stay. A few hours later her daughter died.

For me, it was devastating to lose her—not only as a doctor whose patient had just passed away but also as the woman that I was, waking up to the reality that many of us encounter in most places in the world. I do not even dare to imagine what it was like for her mother, losing her little girl prematurely and unnecessarily. After this tragedy, the mother packed her few belongings and left the hospital without a word, with what I thought was a sacred, sad dignity. She seemed to be resigned, thinking, "Why bother? Why try? What's the point in building hope that life will be better for my children than it was for me?"

Many questions were still left with me: "Was there anything I missed?" "Anything at all that could have saved her?" I thought that I would find answers through experience, but the reality is that seven years of working with MSF only provided more and more unanswered questions. If safe abortion services were available to this girl, she would now be 21 years old. Yet termination of pregnancy on request is forbidden not only in Liberia but also in the vast majority of countries in the world.

Lesson 2: How Did It Come to This?

Rutshuru is a little village in North Kivu, in eastern Democratic Republic of the Congo (DRC). The people of the DRC have been through constant war—as far back as several generations can remember. MSF has worked there providing care for obstetric emergencies and victims of sexual violence. For me, Rutshuru was a place where women came from far away, with all sorts of obstetric complications, traveling on top of a truck or on a motorbike tied with a rope to the driver to avoid falling off when losing consciousness.

Rutshuru presented the unexpected challenge of having to work with women and girl victims of sexual violence. I treated them and signed their medical certificates, so I got to know the stories of how they were attacked while working in the fields, on their way home, or while sleeping at night next to their children.

One story reappears frequently in my thoughts: a 14-year-old girl whose own girlfriends locked her inside a house with the man that was waiting there to rape her. This story hit me hard, broke something inside me, disassembled me. I was shocked not only that the majority of women in the region have been or will be victims of sexual abuse, but also that it was absolutely accepted, to the point that your own girlfriends—those supposedly there for you to call to for help, those meant to protect you, those meant to grieve with you when something like this happens—were the ones setting it up. What had happened to them? How and when did they turn into this? How on earth can a human get rid of empathy in such a clean-stroke way? And, most importantly, can compassion ever be switched on again?

All those women and girls being abused, those being kidnapped for months by soldiers, how do they come back from that dark land? How do they manage life afterward? Living, not merely surviving.

Congolese women and girls are some of my personal heroes, the best example of how wrong this world has gone and how, despite the difficult life they experience every day, they manage to be joyful, warm, strong, funny, and beautiful. They overcome where I would simply have surrendered.

I felt my heart broken, fixed, beating, and expanded about a million times. I remember how I used to dream of digging a tunnel that could get all of the women away from there, to a much better place, where they could just be, without fear. For the first time, and since then, I recognized my new sisters, my daughters, and my mothers.

Lesson 3: The Overwhelming Bright Side

She was too young. She was one of those with a T-shirt with multiple holes, feet covered in dried blood, who had been having contractions since who knows when, at home. She arrived at our little hospital in the west of Côte d'Ivoire. It was her first pregnancy. She was in a critical state.

The baby was dead. Her uterus was clearly ruptured, and she had lost a great deal of blood. A cesarean section was needed to remove the baby and repair her uterus. I explained to her relatives the bad prognosis. We then went to the OR.

In this case, not only was her uterus ruptured but so was her bladder. The tissues were severely damaged after all those hours of being compressed by the baby's head, which could not make its way out. After a long surgical operation, we finally emerged from the OR. It was late, in the middle of the night.

Several female relatives were waiting outside to be informed about her condition. When I told them that she was alive but with a guarded prognosis, the unexpected happened: they started to dance, to sing, to laugh. They grabbed my hands and made me dance to celebrate that she was alive, that she still had a chance where they thought there was already none. I have never felt so much gratitude, so many levels of joy.

She ended up having several abdominal operations for subsequent complications. She also developed a vesico-vaginal fistula: a communication between the bladder and the vagina that produces a constant leaking of urine through the vagina and necessitated complex surgery later on. This condition is considered a curse in many places in the world, leading often to rejection by a husband or partner, expulsion from one's home and village, and all sorts of denigrating treatment within a victim's community. (For more details, see Chapter 10.)

But this girl had a young husband who did not move from the hospital during the 10 days that she was admitted. He was only a boy but one who learned how to do the abdominal dressing she required, a boy who somehow restored a bit of my faith in human beings. I remember his bare, dirty, tired feet next to her bed.

In all my years working with MSF there have been many other countries, patients, lessons learned, colleagues, and impossible diseases. Every country, every patient allowed me to discover a different truth, a different depth to the art of medicine and the dimensions of human suffering. Many times I have wondered about the real effect of what we do, and many times I have only been able to see a benefit for my own personal growth as a human being or as a doctor.

I confess that at some point I believed that not knowing what is happening in the world must be a blissful state. But I have also enjoyed some of the exclusive privileges of being exposed to it: the pure joy and amazement of seeing patients finally improving against all odds, moving further away from the line that divides life and death. At times I laughed with them about how close they were to the other side. I was even upset at them for being so sick, or not knowing what their condition was.

My professional life has acquired a totally different dimension: the duty of being the best possible, with the responsibility of being the only one that might know the solution, the treatment, the diagnosis for the most unlikely condition or disease. In the locations where I have worked, these women have nothing, yet they deserve the finest treatment, the best doctors. So the final question is, "Am I?"

In these settings, one wants to do not only the healing but anything possible to make people's lives a little bit better. One wants desperately to push and force the positive side of the balance through hugs, kisses, smiles, or just cleaning the blood that runs down their legs and saying, "Everything will be all right," in whatever language.

These new experiences changed my landmarks, my scales, and my sensitivity. I am profoundly touched every time a patient says thank you. It sounds both purely unjust and beautiful being thanked when it should be the other way around. How many times did I think, "It is the whole world who thanks you for being this strong and courageous, for carrying the weight of everyone's indifference on your shoulders"? These patients made me understand the magic of healing, the honor of being part of people's hardest and most vulnerable moments in life.

I have welcomed babies in many different countries. I have held the first few seconds of life of hundreds of brand new, warm human beings while wishing them an unlikely good life. I believe this must be one of the most rewarding experiences in the entire world. But as well, my eyes have gotten tired of being opened wide. I have seen many countries, many cultures, many languages, many realities, and one common hub: women suffering, fighting, hoping, helping, carrying on, and trying to make a better future for themselves and their families; women and girls sleeping under a mango tree in a hospital, taking care of their children, sisters, husbands, and mothers; women sleeping in the corridors and being woken when the trolley has to pass on its way to the OR, at any time in the night.

"I am 20 years old. I was raped months ago and I just discovered I am pregnant. If my brothers get to know about this, they will kill me or make me marry the rapist. Can you please help me?"

Why does the world have to be like this?

Maria "Tane" Pilar Luna, MD, is an obstetrician/gynecologist. Since 2008 she has worked with Médecins Sans Frontières (MSF) in Afghanistan, Côte d'Ivoire, Democratic Republic of the Congo, Liberia, Nigeria, Pakistan, Sri Lanka, and Yemen.

ADDITIONAL READING

Anderson FWJ, Morton SU, Naik S, Gebrian B. Maternal mortality and the consequences on infant and child survival in rural Haiti. *Matern Child Health J* (2007) 11:395–401.

Prata N, Sreenivas A, et al. Saving maternal lives in resource-poor settings: facing reality. *Health Policy* 89, no. 2 (Feb. 2009): 131–148.

Sedgh G, et al. Induced abortion: incidence and trends worldwide from 1995 to 2008. *Lancet* 379 (2012): 625–632.

II SURGICAL CARE PRINCIPLES

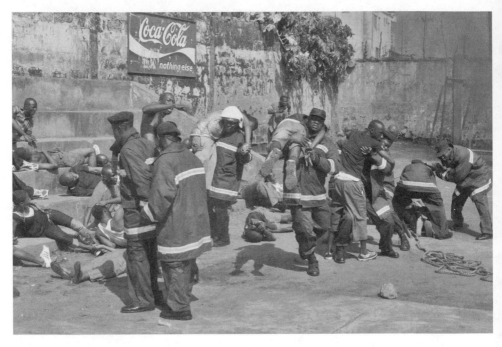

5.1. Mass casualty incident drill, Freetown, Sierra Leone. Photo courtesy T. Peter Kingham

5

Triage and Training

A Mass Casualty Incident Exercise

in Sierra Leone

LUCAS C. CARLSON, MD, MPH, THAIM B. KAMARA, MBBS, FWACS, AND T. PETER KINGHAM, MD, FACS

In memory of Tom T. Rogers, MD, FWACS, trauma surgeon at Connaught Hospital in Freetown, Sierra Leone. He participated in the care of many injured patients and was a strong supporter of mass casualty incident training. He died in 2014 from Ebola.

In March 2009, a leaking oil pipeline exploded and killed scores of people in Freetown, the capital of Sierra Leone. Reportedly, when the leak started, many nearby residents rushed to the scene with buckets to collect oil for their own use. The police were called and ordered the growing crowd back, but their commands went unheeded. Tear gas was used to disperse the crowd but ignited the oil. A massive explosion ensued.

When the flames abated and the smoke cleared, approximately 40 victims were dead on the scene and another 40 were severely burned. The injured victims, with full thickness burns to their faces, bodies, and extremities were brought to Connaught Hospital, the main health facility in the city. The scene was chaotic and the habitually overwhelmed health system was inundated with critically ill patients. Many of the injured died. (For more details on burns, see Chapter 7.)

The magnitude of the tragedy shocked the public. Subsequently, the president of Sierra Leone ordered the Office of Emergency Management and the Ministry of Health and Sanitation to address the shortcomings. Other mass casualty incidents (MCIs) had also recently occurred: a number of multivehicle crashes and a stampede at the football stadium. The need

Table 5.1. Types of mass casualty incidents

Man-made disasters	Natural disasters
Transportation	Earthquake
Industrial	Tsunami
Building collapse or explosion	Hurricane/typhoon
Poisonings (e.g., restaurant or water supply)	Windstorm/tornado
Infectious disease outbreak	Flooding
Active shooter	Forest fire
Terrorist attack	

for a national mass casualty plan and training was recognized and there was now the political will for change.

Unlike conflict, which has a political component and usually begins gradually, disasters mostly strike without warning. Health systems in both conflict and disaster situations are characterized by limited resources and wounded patients requiring surgical care. A number of basic principles such as triage help to reduce the number of deaths and limit disability. Occurring in the context of both conflict and disaster, MCIs are defined as acute events resulting in a large enough number of victims "to disrupt the normal course of emergency and health care services." MCIs are broadly categorized as man-made or natural and can occur either during peacetime or war. These incidents range in size from relatively small events, such as multivehicle crashes, to building collapses, pipeline explosions, and stadium stampedes, to massive disasters such as earthquakes or tsunamis. Although MCIs portrayed in the media typically have hundreds or thousands of victims, most MCIs are much smaller in scale with few victims.

The first step in an MCI response occurs well before the actual event. Development of a general emergency management plan is essential. This is true at a national, regional, local, or even facility level. Although the events causing MCIs vary, the necessary elements of an effective emergency management response are uniform and defined by the "all-hazards model." The principles are: clear lines of responsibility; scalability; whole-of-health multisectorial coordination; and local solutions.

Ideal emergency management plans should: (1) establish clear roles and a command structure; (2) be deployable for small and large emergencies alike; (3) address all components of a victim's health; (4) comprehensively incorporate components of a response including government, healthcare workers, and communication systems; and (5) be initiated from the community level. Developing and maintaining an emergency management plan with each of these elements requires dynamic and interdisciplinary preparation. However, the order created by such a system is invaluable during crisis.

Because of the large number of players involved in any response, a central body should establish the hierarchy and top leadership. National bodies can also establish guidelines and protocols and help direct larger MCI response preparation. These guidelines delineate roles and responsibilities at the facility, community, regional, national, and international levels. An effective MCI response, however, must be initiated and implemented locally. This is imperative because 80% of MCI fatalities occur within the first 20 minutes. Follow-on assistance and resources, such as outside or foreign medical teams, can take days or weeks to mobilize, much too late to prevent these initial deaths.

The three major elements of an MCI response are triage, transport, and treatment. These are also applicable to managing victims wounded in conflict settings or to functioning in a resource-limited environment in general. Triage is derived from the French word "trier," meaning "to sort." It is the practice of dividing victims of MCIs into categories based on degree of injury and whether or not they require immediate medical attention. Traditionally, victims were coded with colored tags:

— Red (Immediate): Life- or limb-threatening injuries requiring immediate attention
— Yellow (Delayed): Requires attention, but no immediate threat to life or limb
— Green (Minor): Minor abrasions or lacerations not requiring immediate attention
— Black (Expectant): Fatal wounds, for palliative care only

The most common protocol for dividing patients into these categories uses the acronym START for "Simple Triage and Rapid Treatment." The first step in this process is to separate the "Greens," the ambulatory victims,

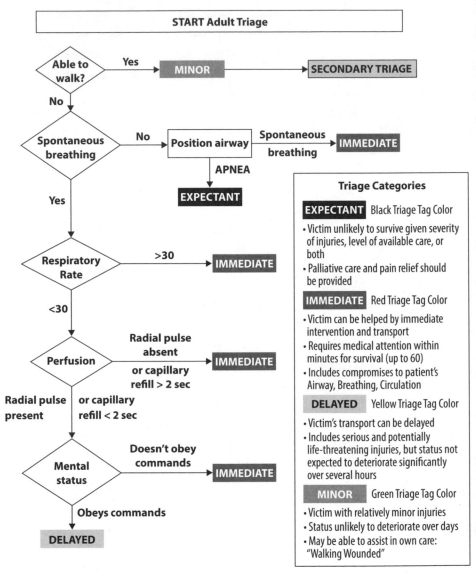

5.2. START: Simple Triage and Rapid Treatment protocol adapted from US Department of Health and Human Services: http://chemm.nlm.nih.gov/startadult.htm

known also as the walking wounded, from the rest. Depending on the size of the event, this is done by simply announcing that all able victims walk to a specific area outside of the immediate incident zone. Then, the remaining victims are categorized as Red, Yellow, or Black by evaluating respiration, pulse rate, and mental status—a process known as the RPM assessment. Those in respiratory distress, having a weak pulse, or with an altered mental status are tagged red. Victims with no pulse and/or no respirations after attempting to open the airway are tagged black. All others are tagged yellow. In the case of unclear decisions, healthcare workers should err on the side of categorizing victims into a more urgent category. For example, if a victim is having substantial difficulty breathing but still has normal mentation, a steady pulse, and fewer than 30 breaths per minute (the cutoff for respiratory distress by the RPM protocol), they could still be tagged red as opposed to yellow.

While actual color-coding of victims may not be feasible in all circumstances, the concept of sorting patients into these categories should be preserved. This is essential because triage allows healthcare workers to effectively and efficiently apply their efforts to doing the greatest good for the greatest number of victims. By definition, resources are scarce in an MCI, and prioritizing treatment in this manner enhances resource allocation and maximizes survival. Also, MCIs are chaotic events. Triage is an objective process that helps to draw order out of the chaos.

Following triage, evaluation is needed to determine where and how to treat the victims. While some victims may require immediate stabilization or be treated on-site, many will require surgery or a higher level of care in a health facility. Unfortunately, there is no established protocol to direct this phase. Healthcare providers can apply emergency training and their medical knowledge to make decisions based on the victim's medical and physiological needs, while considering local context and available resources. Victims are then transported and treated accordingly if higher levels of care are available.

Injuries are not the only concern during an MCI. Other important factors to consider include

- Environmental health: Events such as a building collapse or hurricanes can result in airborne toxin exposure or water supply contamination.

- Chronic diseases: Obesity, heart disease, and diabetes add layers of complexity to treatment of the injured.
- Maternal and child health: Children and pregnant women may require specialized pediatrics or obstetric care.
- Communicable diseases: Unburied corpses do not pose an infectious risk, but crowded health facilities and close living quarters may spread disease.
- Nutrition: Malnutrition impairs wound healing and increases disease susceptibility.
- Healthcare system: Damaged infrastructure and equipment, limited supplies, and incapacitated health personnel may require alternative options to provide adequate care.

While the latter two steps in MCI response, transportation and treatment, are largely dependent on healthcare system capacity before and at the time of the event, START triage is unique to the response process. Regular practice and simulations are essential to ensure that the system functions adequately and responders understand their roles in reacting to unanticipated MCIs.

To train, MCI response can be simulated in a number of ways. It can be discussed and reasoned through in a classroom or seminar format, sometimes called a tabletop exercise. Also MCI responses can be virtually simulated via computer models. The most effective way, however, is physical simulation. The aim of such an exercise is to replicate an MCI in the most accurate way possible. Scenes are set up to resemble the chaotic environment of an MCI, often with appropriate visual distracters, such as burning tires. Then, actors are used to fill the roles of victims and are individually ascribed specific vital signs and scripts for their roles. Responders and healthcare personnel are brought to the scene, where they practice triage, transport, and treatment using real-world scenarios. Afterward, the teams meet to debrief and review the response.

The goals of these exercises are to practice protocols and roles, build teamwork skills, improve communication, and troubleshoot problems within the response plan. The debriefing process is instrumental in achieving these goals and allows responders to explore problems or potential issues with a response plan before an MCI is encountered.

Such an exercise was conducted in Sierra Leone in mid-2009. Surgeons OverSeas (SOS) a US-based nongovernmental organization with a strong relationship to surgeons at Connaught Hospital and with the Ministry of Health and Sanitation helped coordinate. A plan was drafted for a two-day MCI training course. The first day began with didactic lectures and then a tabletop exercise. The second day was a full citywide exercise where more than 180 representatives from the army, police, fire brigade, Office of Emergency Management, Ministry of Health and Sanitation, Red Cross, and the United Nations all worked together to simulate and practice responding in the event of a real disaster.

Thirty medical students were recruited and given scripts for types of injuries that they would have sustained in the event of a massive explosion at a local stadium. When the exercise began, old tires were set on fire, and masses of onlookers were encouraged to storm the police barricades. The fire brigade put out the fire and the local Red Cross assisted with triaging the student actors on the scene. Buses and vehicles transported the "injured" to Connaught Hospital, where stations were established to handle the influx of casualties and "care" was administered. The exercise was regarded as highly effective, highlighted deficiencies and places for improvement, and helped personnel from various sectors organize better communications and chains of command.

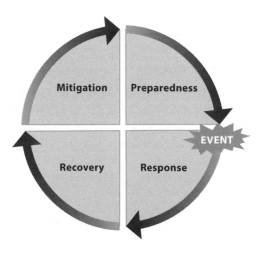

5.3. Disaster management cycle

Development and practice of a response plan is not the end of the preparation phase. As illustrated in Sierra Leone, encountering an MCI can be the key motivation for revamping and redesigning a community's response plan. Similar to MCI simulation, the response team should meet to debrief and review the MCI response after an actual event. This is done to identify system strengths and weaknesses and to learn from mistakes, following the emergency response cycle: Preparedness, Response, Recovery, and Mitigation. MCI response is a rapidly evolving discipline, and it is through this dynamic, cyclical process that systems will continue to improve.

MCIs are universally tragic events, but an effective, disciplined response mitigates their impact. Response comes from the community, but preparation efforts require national involvement, resource allocation, and planning. As the nature of these events increases in severity with the escalating risk factors of climate change, urbanization, and the increasingly complex global political environment, strong response systems will become even more important to ensuring a population's health and resilience.

Thaim B. Kamara, MBBS, FWACS, is Chief of Surgery and Hospital Care Manager at Connaught Hospital in Sierra Leone. He was involved in the initial oil pipeline explosion and the mass casualty incident exercise. T. Peter Kingham, MD, FACS, is President of Surgeons OverSeas (SOS) and an attending surgeon at the Memorial Sloan Kettering Cancer Center in New York, USA. He helped organize and facilitate the mass casualty incident exercise in Sierra Leone.

ADDITIONAL READING

Carlson LC, Hirshon JM, Calvello EJ, Pollak AN. Operative care after the Haiti 2010 earthquake: implications for post-disaster definitive care. *Am J Emerg Med.* 2013 Feb;31(2):429–31.

Geiling J, Burkle FM Jr, Amundson D, Dominguez-Cherit G, Gomersall CD, et al. Resource poor settings: infrastructure and capacity building: care of the critically ill and injured during pandemics and disasters: CHEST consensus statement. *Chest.* 2014 Aug 21. doi: 10.1378/chest.14–0744.

Leow JJ, Brundage SI, Kushner AL, Kamara TB, Hanciles E, Muana A, Kamara MM, Daoh KS, Kingham TP. Mass casualty incident training in a resource-limited environment. *Br J Surg.* 2012 Mar;99(3):356–61.

Levi L, Michaelson M, Admi H, Bregman D, Bar-Nahor R. National strategy for mass casualty situations and its effects on the hospital. *Prehosp Disaster Med.* 2002 Jan–Mar;17(1):12–16.

Risavi BL, Salen PN, Heller MB, Arcona S. A two-hour intervention using START improves prehospital triage of mass casualty incidents. *Prehosp Emerg Care*. 2001 Apr–Jun;5(2):197–9.

Singer AJ, Singer AH, Halperin P, Kaspi G, Assaf J. Medical lessons from terror attacks in Israel. *J Emerg Med*. 2007 Jan;32(1):87–92.

Walls RM, Zinner MJ. The Boston Marathon response: why did it work so well? *JAMA*. 2013 Jun 19;309(23):2441–2.

World Health Organization. *Mass casualty management systems: strategies and guidelines for building health sector capacity*. World Health Organization. 2007. Available from *http://www.who.int/hac/techguidance/MCM_guidelines_inside_final.pdf* (accessed March 5, 2016).

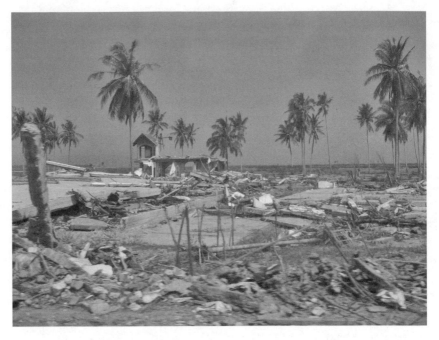

6.1. Banda Aceh after the Indian Ocean earthquake and tsunami. Photo courtesy Adam L. Kushner

6

Wounds and Fractures

Orthopedics after the Indian Ocean Earthquake
and Tsunami

DATTESH R. DAVE, MD, MSC, AND

RICHARD A. GOSSELIN, MD, MPH, MSC, FRCS(C)

Rubble from the earthquake and subsequent tsunami trapped the man's lower leg. Eventually help arrived to free him, but there was no first aid. Four days later, hungry, tired, and having traveled over obliterated roads and through utter devastation, he arrived at the field hospital in Langsa City, Indonesia. He had a fever and an open fracture—his tibia and fibula were broken. His leg was swollen and the wound was infected. For treatment, his wounds were debrided, he was given antibiotics, and an external fixator stabilized his leg. Three days later his fever subsided, the infection improved, and he was stable enough for transfer to Medan, the capital city of Sumatra, for more definitive care. This case, like so many others, was typical after the 2004 Indian Ocean earthquake and tsunami. If victims survived the initial events, they frequently had open fractures that got infected. With a devastated health system and limited resources, simple treatment and temporizing procedures were all that were available and warranted.

Although no official tally exists, it is estimated that more than 220,000 people died as a result of the earthquake and tsunami. The force of the quake and subsequent waves caused widespread destruction to towns and cities along the coast of India, Sri Lanka, Thailand, and especially Indonesia. Some of the worst devastation was to the city of Banda Aceh, the capital of Aceh Province on the Indonesian island of Sumatra. In the city alone, 75% of healthcare workers were killed or displaced, and 17% of the population died or went missing. Of the survivors, 8.5% were injured, with 15% left permanently disabled.

A cross-sectional community survey estimated the overall death and injury rates for Aceh Province at 23.6% and 8.5%, respectively. Women were more likely to die, and men were more likely to be injured. Injuries were most frequent among those aged 20 to 39 years, while death was highest for children under 10 years and the elderly over 60 years. The majority of injured went to a clinic for treatment (63%), but only 14% needed hospitalization. Twenty-one percent of injured victims reported receiving no care.

As medical teams arrived in the days and weeks following the disaster, they were faced with an unusable local infrastructure. Even a week after the initial earthquake, much of Aceh Province was under water. Field hospitals were set up to deal with the injured; however, typical to tsunamis, there were fewer injured compared with the number of deaths. Many of the victims were either killed immediately or swept out to sea. The injured who did gradually begin to arrive for medical attention did so slowly because of the damaged road and transport system. During those first few days and weeks, the orthopedic cases that arrived included contaminated wounds, closed and open fractures, and mangled extremities.

A typical day in a field hospital would consist of morning rounds, debriding wounds, and casting wrist and forearm fractures: all relatively minor procedures. Occasionally external fixation was used to stabilize a fracture, or an amputation performed. The key lesson was that with a combination of massive infrastructure damage, lack of orthopedic hardware, and devastating initial mortality, advanced orthopedic support was nearly impossible locally. Large-scale international support, as exemplified by the USNS *Mercy*, however, was particularly beneficial in this situation.

As part of the international relief effort for the tsunami response, the US government sent the USNS *Mercy*, a naval hospital ship, to the region. The *Mercy* has two main missions: medical and surgical assistance to the branches of the US military, and medical services for humanitarian assistance and disaster relief. The ship's first humanitarian mission was in the Philippines in 1987. The ship was also deployed during the Gulf War in 1990. It subsequently remained stationed in San Diego until the 2004 tsunami.

Over the course of the *Mercy*'s mission off the coast of Banda Aceh, the ship received 75 orthopedic referrals, of which 40 patients were managed surgically. Two categories of injuries were reported: neglected fractures or dislocations, and soft-tissue wounds. The cases presented, on average, 54 days after the time of injury. Overall, 120 orthopedic procedures were performed, including 50 wound debridements, 21 open reduction and internal fixations, 17 intramedullary nail insertions, 7 amputations, and 5 closed reductions.

The *Mercy* reported several clinical and logistical challenges, which were common throughout the relief effort. Of particular concern was the compromised health and overall poor physical condition of many of the patients. The patients also presented with chronic diseases and co-morbidities including diabetes mellitus, hypertension, coronary artery disease, tuberculosis, malnutrition, and anemia. These clinical challenges highlight the importance of partnership and collaboration between surgeons and physicians in disaster management.

Due to the sudden onset of natural disasters, the majority of deaths and injuries occur at the beginning. Initial mortality is typically caused by severe head, chest, and abdominal trauma, while later infectious complications produce the greatest mortality. Survivors and wounded tend to congregate in areas considered safe: remaining functional health facilities, high ground, and open spaces such as stadia or parking lots. Those surviving most commonly suffer musculoskeletal injuries such as soft-tissue wounds, fractures/dislocations, and crush injuries—particularly to the lower extremities. Children and the elderly are particularly vulnerable.

Based on experience from many natural disasters, including the aftermath of the Indian Ocean earthquake and tsunami, the following are some basic technical principles important to save lives and limit disability.

Wounds

All wounds must be considered contaminated and, therefore, not immediately closed. When wounds are closed inappropriately, they often become infected and need to be opened and revised. The most appropriate management of neglected wounds includes the following:

- Washing with clean water (potable but not sterile)
- Sharp debridement (cutting away of dead and diseased tissue)
- Splinting if necessary
- Never suturing closed on initial inspection
- Closing clean wounds after five to seven days

- Using skin grafts or flaps if necessary
- Documenting patient care (possibly writing orders on casts and bandages)
- Tetanus prophylaxis and appropriate antibiotics

Fractures

The most common orthopedic injuries after a natural disaster are fractures. Delayed presentation complicates care as wounds are infected. They initially require serial debridement and broad-spectrum antibiotics. After a wound is clean, flaps, skin grafts, or intramedullary nails may be needed. General principles of fracture management in a conflict or disaster setting include

- Never open a closed fracture
- Never immediately close an open fracture
- Debride open fractures and stabilize with splints, casts, traction, or external fixation
- Primary internal fixation is never indicated, except possibly for hand or foot fractures
- Skeletal traction is useful for hip, femoral shaft, or complex lower extremity fractures
- A sheet or towel may help stabilize a pelvic fracture
- Crush injuries 18 to 24 hours old may require and benefit from open decompression (fasciotomy)
- Crush injuries greater than 24 hours old have greater risk of infection and amputation so should not do fasciotomy but plan for a late reconstruction
- Crush syndrome results in breakdown of dead muscle, electrolyte abnormalities, and kidney problems
- Adequate and appropriate anesthesia is essential, even for simple dressing changes
- Initial stabilization and management are essential for transfer to higher level of care
- Delay definitive management (internal fixation) until appropriate surgical environment, equipment, and supplies are available. After a natural disaster this may be 10 to 14 days.

Amputations

Amputations are common after disasters. Infected or mangled extremities that cannot be saved must be carefully inspected and appropriate principles applied:

- Remove all diseased tissue, but not more than is needed
- Below-knee amputations are preferable to above-knee amputations
- Sites can always be revised to a higher level, especially for an upper extremity
- Stumps primarily left open
- Delayed closure in four to six days if wound is clean
- Create flaps and avoid guillotine amputation, as they always require revision
- Hand injuries appear worse than they are; conserve length and especially the thumb
- For foot amputations, aim to keep the heel and heel pad if possible

Providing orthopedic care after a natural disaster requires a stable infrastructure, reliable orthopedic equipment and supplies, and skilled healthcare personnel. After the tsunami, Indonesian orthopedic surgeons called for donations of equipment such as plates, screws, nails, and external fixators. Local supplies were in short supply, in part, because suppliers did not maintain large stocks. Orthopedic procedures routinely cost US$700, which was too expensive for most of the population, given the annual per capita health expenditure of only US$110. In addition, locally sourced hardware was not universally trusted, due to a lack of testing standards. Donated supplies, including collected plates and screws, could not meet the demand or were caught in the logistic logjam that typically follows a major natural disaster. Additionally, there was a hesitation to rely on used orthopedic hardware. Although sterilization processes existed, there was significant uncertainty about their use in an environment already fraught with contaminated wounds.

Depending on the magnitude and locality of a natural disaster, massive destruction of infrastructure and local capacity may completely render any first response ineffective, particularly in already resource-poor environments. This was certainly the case in Aceh. Relief teams need to prioritize: establish a chain of command; open supply routes; reestablish reliable power, communications, security, water and sanitation; and provide food and shelter for the survivors. The Community needs Assessment for Public health Emergency Response (CASPER) tool is a validated assessment, monitoring, and evaluation method useful during natural disasters, and particularly useful in austere environments.

Once the priorities of chain of command and logistics are established, attention can be turned toward search and rescue, basic first aid, and sorting the injured. Similar to conflict, triage is vital for any disaster or mass casualty event. (For a more detailed discussion of triage, see Chapter 5.) Treatment priorities must be established and scarce resources conserved. The principle is to do the best for the most while keeping those who are beyond saving comfortable.

Life- and limb-saving procedures need to be performed later at better-equipped centers. When there are scores of patients waiting for care, a 10-minute open amputation is preferable to a 4-hour complex limb-saving procedure. Treatment needs to be simple and efficient.

Orthopedic injuries are very common after natural disasters. Although orthopedic surgeons are often among the first international volunteers to assist, there are definite limitations to the type of care that can be administered. When health systems are disrupted and infrastructure destroyed, only limited care can be given. Despite these limitations there is much that can be accomplished by experienced orthopedic surgeons or even minimally skilled health workers with basic supplies and simple equipment. By following prescribed principles, lives can be saved and disability limited.

Richard A. Gosselin, MD, MPH, MSC, FRCS(C), is an orthopedic surgeon. He has extensive experience working in conflict, postconflict, and disaster settings. In January 2004 he spent three weeks as a volunteer after the tsunami in Banda Aceh, Indonesia.

ADDITIONAL READING

Centers for Disease Control and Prevention (CDC). Assessment of health-related needs after tsunami and earthquake—three districts, Aceh Province, Indonesia, 2005. *Morb Mortal Wkly Rep.* 2006, 55(4):93–7.

Dewo P, Magetsari R, Busscher HJ, et al. Treating natural disaster victims is dealing with shortages: an orthopaedics perspective. *Technol Health Care.* 2008;16(4):255–9.

Doocy S, Robinson C, Moodie C, Burnham G. Tsunami-related injury in Aceh Province, Indonesia. *Glob Public Health.* 2009;4(2):205–14.

Gosselin RA. War injuries, trauma and disaster relief. *Techniques in Orthopedics*, 20(2): 97–108, 2005.

Grissom CK. Lessons learned from avalanche survival patterns. *CMAJ*. 2011, 183(7):E366–7.

Millie M, Senkowski C, Stuart L, Davis F, et al. Tornado disaster in rural Georgia: triage response, injury patterns, lessons learned. *Am J Surg*. 2000, 66(3):223–8.

Noe RS, Schnall AH, Wolkin AF, Podgornik MN, et al. Disaster-related injuries and illnesses treated by American Red Cross disaster health services during Hurricanes Gustav and Ike. *South Med J*. 2013, 106(1):102–8.

Prasartritha T, Tungsiripat R, Warachit P. The revisit of 2004 tsunami in Thailand: characteristics of wounds. *Int Wound J*. 2008 Mar;5(1):8–19.

Sechriest VF 2nd, Lhowe DW. Orthopaedic care aboard the USNS Mercy during, Operation Unified Assistance after the 2004 Asian tsunami: a case series. *J Bone Joint Surg Am*. 2008 Apr;90(4):849–61.

Uscher-Pines L, Vernick JS, Curriero F, Lieberman R, Burke TA: Disaster-related injuries in the period of recovery: the effect of prolonged displacement on risk of injury in older adults. *J Trauma*. 2009, 67(4):834–40.

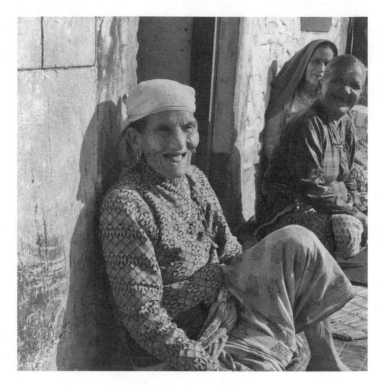

7.1. Elderly woman in Nepal. Photo courtesy Shailvi Gupta

Burn Care

Experience from the Nepalese Civil War

BARCLAY T. STEWART, MD, MSCPH, AND
BRIJESH MISHRA, MS, MCH

A 5-year-old Nepali boy and his family, exhausted from days of retreating into the Himalaya Mountains, fell asleep next to a makeshift stove to keep warm. In the night, the boy's clothes caught fire. Although his parents immediately extinguished the flames, he had already suffered deep burns over the areas once covered by his clothes. His father wrapped him in a blanket and carried him for several days before they reached a road and joined a bus that would carry them to the hospital. When they finally arrived, the boy was gasping quietly for air. His father was exhausted and desperate. We laid the boy down on a stretcher and unwrapped him, exposing the wet soot on his charred body that smelled like smoke and pus. He stared beyond us and never made a sound as we worked to set an intravenous catheter and determine how severe his burn was. Nearly 70% of his body surface area was burned; most of that was deep and infected from the days of travel before reaching care. We kept him warm and hydrated and gave pain medication to keep him comfortable. He died soon thereafter with his father at his side quietly chanting a prayer. There was no way to save him—not there, not then.

From 1996 to 2006, the Nepalese Civil War was fought between government forces and Maoist fighters; the conflict resulted in an estimated 20,000 deaths. In addition to those killed from direct conflict, the fighting also destabilized the healthcare system and resulted in many more preventable deaths and disabilities. In Nepal, burns were the second most common cause of injury before the war. During the conflict, the numbers of burn patients soared, usually the result of homemade roadside explosives, bottled petrol bombs, and the breakdown of safe infrastructure.

Nearly 90% of burns around the world occur in developing countries. People living in low-income countries suffer disproportionately for a number of reasons: the use of open cooking fires, inflammable fabrics, and loose fitting clothing such as saris in South Asia; the limited use of smoke detectors; unsupervised children cooking or caring for younger siblings; paraffin stoves are used for heating; and fuel safety measures are inadequate. Compounding the greater incidence of burns in developing countries is the limited ability of healthcare systems to care for patients with complex needs, such as those with burn injury.

In high-income countries, burn care is frequently provided at specialized centers and includes rapid and efficient prehospital services, timely resuscitation, critical care, early burn excision and grafting, physical therapy, and rehabilitation. Such capacity is almost uniformly absent in low-resource settings. Optimal burn care requires many resources: large amounts of sterile gauze and bandages, functioning operating rooms, blood banks, and skilled personnel. During conflict, when health systems are disrupted and supplies are in even shorter supply, optimal burn care is impossible; however, if the basic principles of triage and war surgery are married with several tenets of burn care, lives can be saved and disabilities reduced.

Unlike household burns, which are caused mostly by flames or scalding, burns during conflict often result from explosives. As with other types of war wounds, these injuries are contaminated from projectiles and shrapnel, as well as the blast itself. In addition, electrical and chemical burns are more common during conflict than peacetime. Exposed wiring in neglected or destroyed infrastructure increases the risk of electrical injury and electrocution. Small external electrical burns often disguise serious underlying injuries and require major surgical debridement. High-voltage electrical injuries can also cause heart rhythm changes, fractures, intestinal perforations, and nerve damage. Chemical weapons are used less frequently in modern conflicts than in times past. Although banned by the 1993 Chemical Weapons Convention, chemical weapon use has not fully ceased, and stockpiles of phosphorus, mustard, and sarin gas still exist. Clinicians working in conflict should be familiar with the effects of these agents in order to recognize and report their use.

Most acute burn care principles are universal: provide fluid resuscitation, adequate nutrition, and physical therapy. Our experience in Nepal taught us three additional lessons: heroic efforts may ultimately lead to greater suffering for patients and families; stoicism should not be interpreted as permission to withhold pain relief; and, there are often various ways to obtain a satisfactory outcome.

As discussed in Chapter 5, appropriate triage of the injured is an important conflict and disaster care principle. Burn patients require a great deal of care; therefore, those who will not survive must be identified early to avoid exhausting scarce resources. Estimating total body surface area (TBSA) with 2nd and 3rd degree burns is an important first step. Those with more than 50% TBSA rarely survive in low-resource settings.

Similarly, patients with smaller burns, but who had inhaled noxious or heated gases, were also at high risk of dying despite maximal care. At our facilities, these patients were given fluids and pain medication for comfort and their families were counseled about the inevitable loss of their loved one.

In cases that were less clear, we would treat aggressively for a short period of time and reassess the patient to determine the prognosis. For example, if a child needed ventilation, he or she was intubated. But since there were no ventilators, family members were taught how to use a bag valve mask and then took turns bagging their child. This would continue for hours or days until a determination was made whether or not the child was improving and had a reasonable chance at meaningful survival. Subjecting patients with large burns to futile care for days or weeks with minimal chance of survival is ultimately inhumane for them and their family. Similarly, attempts at heroic care can consume resources without benefit and imperil patients who otherwise might live. Thoughtful and realistic triage is key to burn care success in low-resource settings.

No matter what part of the body is burned, fluid loss and inappropriate tissue swelling is the hallmark of a burn injury. Ensuring brisk, appropriate fluid resuscitation is imperative to avoid worsening injury and life-threatening dehydration. However, overresuscitation also has negative consequences and can consume excess resources. In many low-income countries, patients present days after a burn due to a number of barriers to care (e.g., cost, poor roads). This is particularly true during times of conflict. Therefore, burn patients usually arrive severely dehydrated. Those who are able to drink arrive in better condition than those who are not able, but then often suffer from infections and malnutrition. For these patients, antibiotics and tetanus vaccines were routinely administered, as many patients were unvaccinated. Local high-protein and high-calorie foods helped with healing. Feeding victims blended food through nasogastric tubes directly into their stomachs often started within the first day to stave off malnutrition. Prior to performing any operation, nutritional status was optimized to avoid complications of nonhealing wounds.

Burn wounds must be properly dressed and done so in a humane way. Except for the deepest injuries, where nerve endings are destroyed, most burns are extremely painful. Therefore, pain management with narcotics or ketamine is essential, especially when changing dressings. Burn wound care requires time, large amounts of gauze and bandages, and human resources. Skilled burn nurses are rare in crisis settings. While some patients attempt to remain calm and dignified during burn dressing changes, surveys of patients after recovery document wound care as the most painful and difficult aspect of their experience. Many of the children we cared for were remarkably calm during wound care; however, such stoicism should not be interpreted as permission to withhold pain medications. To ensure adequate pain relief and compensate for the lack of nursing care, sizable dressing changes are preferably done in the operating room with anesthesia. This is commonplace in low-resource crisis settings; burns often comprise between 10% to 25% of all procedures performed in an operating theater during humanitarian surgery assistance.

As part of optimal management, well-resourced burn centers perform early surgical excision and grafting of wounds unlikely to heal within a few weeks. Early excision reduces the length of time patients sit with open wounds and limits aggressive scarring, which can be disfiguring and can lead to contractures and loss of function. In low-resource settings, excision is not always possible; fortunately, many burns can be allowed to simply heal for up to six weeks. Though often difficult for medical personnel from high-income countries to adopt, in appropriately selected patients this nonoperative technique can result in satisfactory outcomes, fewer overall procedures, and lower consumption of supplies. As with any intervention, the surgical team must consider the skills and services provided at their facility before deciding to operate. For instance, excision of burns can be extremely bloody. Without the capacity for blood transfusion and skilled anesthesia, decisions to excise a significantly sized burn should not be made lightly.

Healing burns, like all scars, contract. Families often do not have the resources to bring a burned child to the hospital immediately after injury. Such wounds are often small or on curious children's hands. Weeks after what seems a small burn, however, the wound contracts and the hand may become nonfunctional. It is then that the patients present to the hospital. Fortunately, severe disability from small burns on hands, feet, and joints can be reduced with relatively simple surgical techniques, even in the most austere settings. Specialized physical therapists who oversee exercises that reduce contractures and make scars more pliable are usually not present. Therefore, healthcare personnel must be well versed in simple splinting and physical therapy routines that can be taught to and monitored by families.

Our facility, like many others in low-resource settings, often lacked even low-cost supplies, such as oxygen, bandages, and splints; narcotics for pain control; and equipment (e.g., beds, diathermy). We often had to improvise. For example, burns to the hands and feet were dressed with an-tibiotic burn cream (i.e., silver sulfadiazine) and placed in plastic bags or surgical gloves and then splinted to avoid using bandages. When this burn cream was absent, a mixture of honey and ghee (i.e., clarified butter) or oil was an effective alternative. If Vaseline-impregnated dressings were not available, fine mesh gauze smeared with petroleum jelly and then sterilized was equally effective. Other locally made dressings have included appropri-ately prepared potato peels or banana leaves.

Burns do not only injure the skin and underlying tissues, nor does care stop once the patient leaves the hospital. Burns are disfiguring and often occur during life-threatening events. Therefore, patients frequently need mental health and social support to prevent or manage depression, anxiety, adjustment or posttraumatic stress disorder. The stigma associated with burn scars can be devastating as patients attempt to retake some control of their life and reintegrate into their community. Mental health disorders and stigma can be as bad as or even more disabling than the burn injury itself. Therefore, efforts to include support for these aspects of burn care should be considered during conflict or a burn-related disaster.

Often forgotten are the extreme stresses that burn care providers deal with when taking care of their patients. This relentlessly intense and emotional work, especially during conflict or disaster, can take a toll on staff morale. Working closely with national staff and sharing in care successes, as well as failures, can alleviate some of the stress and help build an effective team.

During conflict, too many victims, such as the Nepali boy we cared for, do not survive their burn injuries. When establishing surgical assistance projects during crisis, planners must consider the equipment, supplies, and personnel needed to care for burn patients. In addition, national support of prevention strategies is essential, as are ensuring sustainable mechanisms for low-cost interventions such as initial wound care, resuscitation, and physical therapy. Furthermore, strengthening healthcare systems so that they can provide prehospital care and have established pathways for referral of those in need of more complex care is important.

Burn care challenges low-resource health systems, providers, and most of all patients and their families. However, burn patients can make extraordinary recoveries when basic principles are followed, even in austere settings.

Barclay Stewart, MD, MscPH, is a general surgical resident at the University of Washington. He spent three months working at Kanti Children's Hospital's burn ward and with burn care outreach teams in 2005. Brijesh Mishra, MS, MCh, is a plastic and reconstructive surgeon now working at King Georges Medical University in India. He spent two years in Nepal working at B.P. Koirala Health Institute caring for acute burns and performing reconstructive burn surgery immediately after the war from 2007.

ADDITIONAL READING

Ahuja RB, Bhattacharya S. Burns in the developing world and burn disasters. *BMJ.* 2004;329(7463):447–9.

Atiyeh BS, Gunn SW, Hayek SN. Military and civilian burn injuries during armed conflicts. *Annals of Burns and Fire Disasters.* 2007;20(4):203–15.

Carlson LC, Rogers TT, Kamara TB, Rybarczyk MM, Leow JJ, Kirsch TD, et al. Petroleum pipeline explosions in sub-Saharan Africa: a comprehensive systematic review of the academic and lay literature. *Burns: journal of the International Society for Burn Injuries.* 2014.

Giannou C, Baldan M. *War surgery: working with limited resources in armed conflict and other situations of violence.* Geneva, Switzerland: International Committee of the Red Cross, 2010.

Gupta S, Wong E, Mahmood U, Charles AG, Nwomeh BC, Kushner AL. Burn management capacity in low and middle-income countries: a systematic review of 458 hospitals across 14 countries. *International journal of surgery*. 2014.

Mishra B, Koirala R, Tripathi N, et al. Plastic surgery—myths and realities in developing countries: experience from eastern Nepal. *Plastic surgery international* 2011; 870902.

Rossi LA, Vila Vda S, Zago MM, Ferreira E. The stigma of burns: perceptions of burned patients' relatives when facing discharge from hospital. *Burns: journal of the International Society for Burn Injuries*. 2005;31(1):37–44.

van Kooij E, Schrever I, Kizito W, Hennaux M, Mugenya G, Otieno E, et al. Responding to major burn disasters in resource-limited settings: lessons learned from an oil tanker explosion in Nakuru, Kenya. *Journal of trauma*. 2011;71(3):573–6.

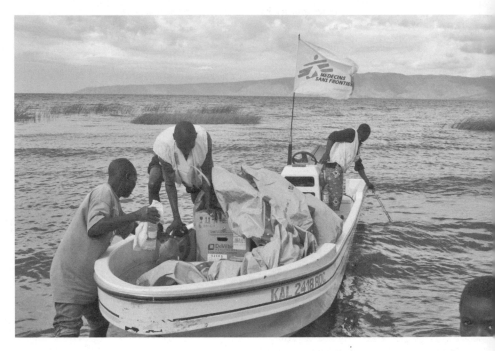

8.1. En route to Baraka, Democratic Republic of the Congo. Photo courtesy Marten van Wijhe

8

Anesthesia

An Assessment Mission in the Congo

MARTEN VAN WIJHE, MD, PHD

"Ai bwana, rudi nyumbani!"—meaning "Sir, return home!"—exclaimed the taxi driver on my way from the airport to the hotel in Kigali, the capital of Rwanda. I had just mentioned my plans to travel to Baraka in South Kivu in the Democratic Republic of the Congo (DRC), and according to him the other side of the Rwanda-DRC border was an unhealthy place to go.

This advice was slightly unsettling. I knew that turmoil and conflict had existed for decades in North and South Kivu, the eastern provinces of the DRC that bordered on the Great Lakes countries of Uganda, Rwanda, Burundi, and Tanzania. My briefing at Médecins Sans Frontières (MSF) headquarters in Amsterdam had covered the unrest caused by Hutu militias that sought refuge in the region after their role in the Rwandan genocide. Conflict between the different factions and local militias, as well as trouble with the Congolese military, led to the establishment of a United Nations peacekeeping force in the area. Local communities were trapped in the middle, and their health and well-being suffered. Despite the unrest, I was assured the situation was relatively calm and it would be an easy trip by plane, taxi, MSF vehicle, and MSF boat to Baraka on the western shore of Lake Tanganyika. My assignment was to assess and report on anesthesia quality at the MSF-supported government hospital.

Anesthesia is the medical specialty that cares for patients before, during, and after surgery. Anesthesia providers administer general or regional anesthesia, monitor patients' vital signs, and share responsibility for patient care and safety with the surgeon. The armamentarium of the modern anesthesiologist to guide clinical decision making and care includes airway control, artificial ventilation, circulatory support, and monitoring equipment. In many conflict and postconflict settings, especially in rural Africa, these items are mostly absent.

What I found in Baraka was quite typical. To support breathing during an operation, instead of an automated anesthesia machine, the surgical team only had a self-inflating balloon with facemasks. Instead of 100% compressed oxygen, only a maximum of 5 liters per minute from an oxygen concentrator could be given. Intravenous fluids, such as Ringer's solution, normal saline, and 5% dextrose were in stock; as were various anesthesia medications, including adrenaline, atropine, diazepam, ketamine, metoclopramide, and tramadol. For spinal anesthesia there was hyperbaric bupivicaine 0.5% and ephedrine. Blood pressure cuffs, stethoscopes, and pulse oximeters were available for monitoring vital signs, and there was a stock of urine collection bags to monitor fluid balance. By rural African standards, Baraka Hospital was well equipped. By European standards it was severely limited. The situation, however, allowed many emergency operations to be performed, though many other procedures were excluded due to a concern about patient safety and mission priorities.

Despite the limitations, many operations were safely performed with MSF providing free emergency care to all in need. More than half of the operations were obstetric emergencies, such as cesarean sections for obstructed labor or procedures to control bleeding before or after delivery. (For more detail on women's health, see Chapters 4 and 9.) Other common emergency operations included laparotomy for intestinal perforation from typhoid fever, intestinal obstructions due to hernia, and management of wounds secondary to violence or road traffic injuries. (For more detail on general procedures, see Chapter 3.) Of the more than 800 procedures in 2013 and 2014, fewer than 30 were for elective indications.

Though sophisticated anesthesia machines were lacking, one drug routinely used to anesthetize patients in Baraka and similar facilities was ketamine. This wondrous medication allows the surgeon to work without causing the patient acute suffering. After ketamine is injected into a patient's veins, it brings on a state of mental oblivion and indifference, and it also diminishes the physiological effects of the surgical trauma. The patients do not feel or realize what is happening, but they still breathe, their heart beats, and their mental functions are temporarily disabled. Ket-

Table 8.1. Major operations performed at Baraka Hospital in 2013 and 2014

Procedure	2013	2014
Cesarean section	606	609
Laparotomy	131	130
Hernia repair	75	85
Other interventions	10	17
Total	822	841

amine allows the surgeon to work reasonably comfortably; however, the patient's muscles are not fully relaxed, in contrast to anesthesia with other more sophisticated means. Providing anesthesia with ketamine is not very complicated—dose by body weight, repeat dosing at regular intervals or when the patient starts to move, though still unaware of the surgery being performed. One must be vigilant. Giving too little results in a patient who moves, making surgery difficult or dangerous; give too much and the patient is anesthetized for longer than necessary. Although ketamine is quite safe to use, it has some limitations. Alcoholic patients are resistant to its effects, and it is unsuitable for eye or brain surgery. Otherwise, it can be safely used on children and even bleeding patients, as it tends to raise blood pressure.

Local infiltration is an alternative when general anesthesia is undesirable or not possible. Inguinal hernia repairs and even cesarean sections may be successfully performed with local infiltration anesthesia. Another effective, but potentially more dangerous alternative, is spinal anesthesia. This form of regional anesthesia was discovered over a century ago. It provides a temporary loss of sensation in the lower half of the body. Dosing is critical; too little does not block pain, but too much can quickly lead to death. Safely administering spinal anesthesia requires greater expertise than ketamine or local infiltration.

Anesthesia providers from high-income countries who volunteer to work in rural African hospitals must be prepared for significantly different conditions from their home environments. At most district hospitals in postconflict or low-level conflict areas, such as in North and South Kivu, infectious diseases form the greatest part of the hospital workload, but surgical cases are plentiful and can be challenging due to late presentation, poor condition of the patients, lack of diagnostics and medications, and limited treatment options. A lack of locally trained medical doctors leads to "task-sharing," whereby nurses or technicians provide surgery or anesthesia. Hospitals' cleanliness is always an issue, and sterility can be difficult to maintain. In Baraka, the operating room doors were hanging off their hinges, the air-conditioning did not work, and there was no running water. The linen and surgical gowns were thin and showed numerous tears and holes, and the operation table was rusted into a solidly fixed position. To provide safe surgical care, MSF standards allow for some flexibility, but surgical mortality must be kept below 1%. This often means that heroic measures or too-complex cases cannot be operated on, as resources are in short supply and staff have limited capabilities.

Aside from the physical resources and technical skills needed to safely anesthetize patients, anesthesia personnel play an important role in data collection. When I visited Baraka as the anesthesia advisor, I was expected to look through the hospital setup and weigh the clinical results as shown by the collected data. These data included the number of patients seen, where they lived, diagnosis, response to treatment, and insights gained in the efficacy of interventions and needs for adjustment.

These data, once collected by the medical team, were then passed on to the medical coordinator (MedCo), the person responsible for health activities in the country based in the provincial capital. The Health Advisor based in Amsterdam also received a copy of the data. The aim of my visit, as the anesthesia advisor, was to assess the conditions but not make judgments based on Western standards. I was not there to compile a lengthy list of shortcomings but rather to appreciate the team's efforts and make simple suggestions on how to improve clinical outcomes. My final report contained a list of simple advice to the MedCo and Health Advisor. My recommendations included ordering equipment, such as more oxygen concentrators, and introducing a new drug, recently added to the MSF catalogue and appropriate for the project.

Advice in such settings is difficult to give. The optimal solution is often known but hardly possible under the circumstances. For example, suggesting hiring more national staff physicians is not realistic when there are so few in the country. Raising the standard of anesthetic care would imply increasing the number of nurses with anesthetic training (three years in DRC). Although ideal, it is not readily possible. Of necessity, nurses without formal anesthesia training provide anesthesia under supervision of the surgeon.

The World Health Organization (WHO) developed a three-level system of classifying health facilities. Health centers (Level 1), district hospitals (Level 2), and referral hospitals (Level 3) are the main types of facilities. Each level is mandated to deliver a certain standard of medical and surgical care administered by competent health professionals. The ideals of the WHO classification are often not met in rural African hospitals such as Baraka. Though not an official level, Level 1.5 becomes a reality in many MSF settings. Such facilities, though lacking all the resources needed for full Level 2 status, undertake operations such as cesarean sections and other emergency operations. Lack of funding by host countries for a strong health system results in poor infrastructure, limited equipment, supplies, and drugs, and inadequate training of healthcare personnel. Though tempting, the solution is not to fly in modern fully equipped hospitals with international expatriate staff but instead to build on what is already locally available, with external assistance where needed.

Volunteer specialists generally come for a few months' work. They need careful briefing on how to prepare and what to expect. One of the difficulties MSF and other international aid organizations encounter is the *inexperience* of Western specialists. This may sound odd, but instead of superspecialists, generalists with a combination of obstetric, general, and trauma surgical skills are required. As such combinations no longer exist in Western medical systems, many volunteer surgeons opt for additional training with colleagues. Well-rounded anesthesiologists are also needed, but they are not as difficult to find.

Emergency medical aid during a time of conflict or disaster is not synonymous with medical development aid. In conflict or disaster situations where mass casualties overwhelm the local health system, or the system itself is partly or wholly destroyed, external medical and logistical staff can help save lives. The aim should be to offer temporary assistance until local authorities can take over again. Medical development aid on the other hand typically takes place in a more stable and controlled setting where a government requests either another government or a nongovernmental organization to assist with training personnel or to deliver limited equipment and supplies. In North and South Kivu the ongoing conflict necessitates that MSF and other groups provide both direct care and invest in longer-term projects, such as infrastructure maintenance and training of personnel.

Although surgeons and emergency operations may garner the most attention during a conflict, providing safe anesthesia is a necessity. The decades-long conflict in the DRC mandates a continuing presence. My visit to Baraka confirmed the hard and conscientious work of the team but also the need for external assessments to provide an outside view to improve the surgical care for the community.

ADDITIONAL READING

Bartholomeusz L, Lees J. *Safe anaesthesia: a training manual where facilities are limited.* 3rd ed., 2006. Available through T.A.L.C. http://www.talcuk.org.

Clyburn P, Collis R, Harries S. *Obstetric anaesthesia for developing countries.* Oxford University Press, 2010.

Dobson MB. *Anaesthesia at the district hospital.* WHO. 2nd ed., 2000.

King M, ed. *Primary anaesthesia.* Oxford University Press, 1990.

Waters DAK, Wilson IH, Leaver RJ, Bagshawe A. *Care of the critically ill patient in the tropics.* Macmillan, 2nd ed., 2004.

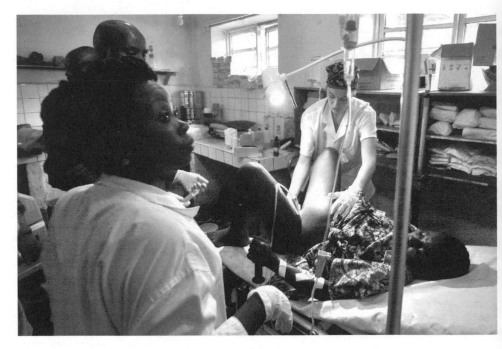

9.1. Labor ward, Democratic Republic of the Congo. Photo courtesy Nick Czernkovich

9

Obstetrics and Gynecology during a Civil War

JUDY M. LEE, MD, MPH, MBA, FACOG

The knock at the door to the compound came in the middle of the night. I reflexively jumped out of bed as the word *"ticket!"*—meaning a new case had arrived to the maternity ward—cut through the silence. I walked to the front gate, chose a bicycle, and quickly pedaled to the hospital. Upon arriving in the maternity ward, I gazed upon the face of a scared woman who was clearly in pain, in tears, but who hardly uttered a whimper. With the help of the midwife, who also assisted in translations during the nights, we diagnosed what was certainly a uterine rupture. We could not get a fetal heart rate and the patient's clinical signs were deteriorating. Already, the ticket to the anesthesiologist had gone out and the operating theater person was on his way to get the generator going. On entering her abdomen through the previous vertical scar, I found a dead fetus and brisk bleeding from her shredded and ruptured uterus. I quickly performed an emergency cesarean hysterectomy. Meanwhile, team members struggled to find blood donors.

Later that day, having finished my mission, I left with this same patient, accompanying her across the front defense line, where she would then proceed on to a government hospital with facilities that could see her through her postoperative course. Her scared face was now one of gratitude, but she had no idea how much of my own thoughts she reflected.

In war zones, few things go according to plan and one can never be fully prepared for their first experience. When one is working abroad in a non-English-speaking country, nonverbal cues and the physical examination become paramount to clinical work. A smile and a hug go a long way in communicating, even more than words. Patients do not present with the usual conditions; ancillary services and support staff are limited or nonexistent; and familiar tools of the trade can be scarce or found lacking altogether. Under these conditions, one has to think outside of the box in more ways than I had ever imagined or experienced. While the mental and physical sacrifices were tough, I found while I was riding in the transport heading home that I was far more grateful for the lessons I learned delivering obstetric and gynecologic care during a civil war and for the people and patients I met.

More importantly perhaps was learning to deal with the vulnerabilities of my patient population and observing how these women were coping with the loss of husbands, children, families, home, and security. Many often sat together in quiet camaraderie in the courtyard, but others would keep to themselves. I do not know what happened to my patients and their babies, but it was a humbling experience watching them walk away from the hospital into an uncertain future and social isolation, where all previously known societal infrastructures had crumbled. I had neither the skills nor the resources to deal with the mental health impact of the ongoing conflict.

My mission did not begin as expected. Convoys through no-man's-land were blocked. So instead of traveling directly to the northern region where I was to work, I waited at the front defense line until the International Committee of the Red Cross could negotiate another agreement for safe passage.

Those days were spent in setting up and staffing makeshift clinics for the many displaced persons around the area. I examined babies, children, and men, in addition to the occasional pregnant woman. With nothing but a stethoscope, antibiotics, and a translator, I diagnosed scabies and upper respiratory and urinary tract infections. It was daunting to be without my usual array of tools, ancillary services, and the familiar context within which I had trained. When patients with a significant clinical finding sat with me at the foldout table, I felt hopeless suggesting they go to the nearest hospital for lab tests or imaging studies. I knew they probably would not go.

At night, the distant and not-so-distant booms from the shelling made the windows and doors rattle. I quickly noticed I was the only one always walking into the main room, prepared to head to the bunker. "Oh, but those were outgoing shells," I was always told in the morning. After three weeks, when the permission to travel was granted, I was outfitted for my trip across the front defense line. I wore an oversized jacket stuffed full with ketamine vials, cheese, and chocolate. The checkpoints and inspections made me uneasy. But I arrived safely and met the team.

The maternity ward had 30 beds and was staffed by four midwives. As is common in such settings, there was no ultrasound, doppler, cardiotocograph, or phototherapy. Intravenous fluids were administered by a drip count per minute. Oxygen cylinders were in limited supply. Three local scrub assistants took turns sleeping at the hospital to cover for emergent cases. A generator was available at night if there was an emergency, but it required waking up a staff member, who then had to find the man with the key.

Because convoys occurred infrequently, we made difficult decisions regarding when to use our increasingly limited resources. The government also restricted or denied certain requests for supplies. I used catgut when we ran out of other, more appropriate sutures. At one point, the rats ate through all the gauze in the storeroom. We traveled into town and tested other material in the autoclave to see what was best for fashioning laparotomy sponges for our surgical cases. At times, we ran out of some essential medicines and could not even treat malaria, one of the most common antenatal conditions. When the compressed oxygen ran low, the pediatrician was forced to choose which neonate needed it most.

For me, the nights were the most stressful. My sleep was fitful, as I uneasily awaited a knock at the compound door and a voice yelling, *"ticket!"* Then I would wake, grab a flashlight, and pedal as fast as I dared on the pockmarked road to the hospital. After the rains, I also had to watch out for snakes along the fence. The kerosene lanterns at the hospital attracted hordes of moths, throwing fleeting shadows as you carried them from one room to the next. Hauntingly, an eerie silence accompanied each emergency. The cases were usually a decreased fetal heart rate, heavy vaginal bleeding from a miscarriage, complications after an attempted abortion, or a problem with a placenta. The midwife on call performed the normal deliveries. There was no blood bank, but many women needed transfusions. The sounds of geckos and other nocturnal creatures were interrupted by the loudspeaker calls urging immediate blood donation.

In the ward, whenever there were more patients than beds, the newly arrived patients would simply sleep under an occupied bed. Without an ultrasound I relied heavily on a physical exam to confirm fetal position or estimate fetal weight. The midwives used the Pinard fetal stethoscope to assess fetal heart rates, equipment which I had only seen pictures of in the historical section of obstetric textbooks. They found my use of the stethoscope to listen to the baby amusing. I could almost hear an older mentor of mine, who said how newer generations are increasingly reliant on technology and are losing the art of clinical examination.

One patient was brought in obtunded, having suffered what sounded like eclampsia. She never recovered. Most cesarean sections were done under spinal anesthesia, and postpartum tubal ligations were done under ketamine. Babies who appeared jaundiced were taken out into the sunlight, as we lacked phototherapy equipment. We made little cardboard beds and eyeshades for them.

In the antenatal and gynecology clinics and on the wards, anemia was assessed either clinically or by the hemoglobin color meter, where blood is obtained by a pinprick, spread on a slide and compared to a color chart. Luckily we had an adequate supply of iron, folic acid, and multivitamins. The most common form of contraception was the Copper T IUD or Depo-Provera injections. Routine screening for breast and cervical cancers was nonexistent. One patient complained of a foul discharge and constant spotting. Her exam revealed a beefy red, fungating mass with areas of necrotic tissue almost replacing the cervix. I could only transfer her on the next convoy out of the region, knowing that her prognosis was poor even if she had been in the United States.

My first several weeks were some of the most physically and psychologically draining weeks of my professional life. Despite the passing months, I could still feel very lonely in my despair at wanting to do more than was possible. My more seasoned teammates were a source of support. We did what we could with what we had, because this was all that was available. That these conditions are routine in conflict instilled in me a deeper respect for those men and women who have lived with or worked in conflict for much of their lives.

Although mental health was important for the team, the impact of conflict affected the patients in dramatic ways. At the time, suicide rates were high. For women, a common form of suicide was overdosing on chloroquine, a medicine used to treat malaria. It was also used to attempt an abortion. One case of suicide involved a woman who doused herself with gasoline and set herself on fire. I can still see how remnants of her melted-on nightgown sloughed away with her skin as we attempted to keep her alive.

We also saw trauma cases resulting from land mines in areas where children played. Some of the antipersonnel land mines were brightly colored, causing a curious child to pick them up. While covering for the general surgeon I had to perform finger amputations and conservatively debride hand injuries. Other trauma cases were caused by accidental gun discharges. Once, when the surgeon had just left on a convoy, I heard shouts from a different part of the hospital, as a young female patient was brought in, having accidentally been shot. As we were rolling her back to the operating room, I examined the entrance wound located near her groin and tracked the bullet into her abdominal cavity. She died before we could even get her onto the operating room table.

Watching the compound get smaller as we drove away, I did not think my last patient realized how grateful I was that she was alive and for the experience of working in an area of conflict. Providing women's health in a war zone was a challenging and unforgettable opportunity. During conflict, the needs of vulnerable populations are often neglected, and the long term mental health outcomes should be addressed in a coordinated effort. However, I learned possibilities do exist for providing care and saving lives. And if nothing could be done, that shared struggle with a patient creates a bond I will never be able to describe and gives me strength to carry on. To quote from a Nobel Peace Prize presentation speech, "To show each victim a human face, by showing respect for his or her dignity, is to create hope for peace and reconciliation."

ADDITIONAL READING

Groen RS, Kushner AL. Obstetrics, in Meara JG, McClain CD, Rogers SO, Mooney DP, eds. *Global surgery and anesthesia manual: providing care in resource-limited settings*, 2014, CRC Press.

King, M. *Primary surgery: non-trauma*, vol. 1, 1990. Oxford University Press.

Lester F, Washington S. Gynecology, in Meara JG, McClain CD, Rogers SO, Mooney DP, eds. *Global surgery and anesthesia manual: providing care in resource-limited settings*, 2014, CRC Press.

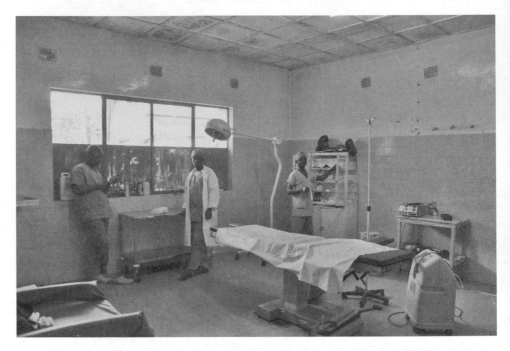

10.1. An operating room in the Democratic Republic of the Congo. Photo courtesy Chiels Liu

Sexual Violence

Genital Fistula and Conflict

LAURI J. ROMANZI, MD, FACOG, FPMRS,
AND EDNA ADAN ISMAIL, SRN, CMB, SCM

Armed rebels invaded the home of a teenage student. Despite her cries and protest, she was sexually assaulted. Her older brother was forced to watch. He tried to protest but was killed. His lifeless body was then placed next to her as the rebels repeatedly raped her, violated her with their weapons, beat her, and then stabbed her multiple times in the abdomen. Though left for dead, she survived the abuse and was later transported for care. Her numerous injuries included a complex genital fistula between her vagina and her urinary and colorectal tracts.

A genital fistula is an abnormal connection between the upper (uterus and cervix) or lower (vagina, perineum) genital tract and the bladder, urethra, ureters, rectum, or anus. Women with a fistula leak urine or stool. Most international efforts addressing this issue focus on obstructed labor, one of the historic causes of genital fistula. Obstructed labor occurs when childbirth lasts two or more days and the baby's head compresses the soft tissue of the mother's genital tract against the maternal pelvic bones, causing necrosis of the soft tissues, resulting in abnormal connections between organ systems.

A traumatic genital fistula occurs when the vaginal walls are perforated from a blunt or penetrating injury or from sexual violence, which may include forced genital insertion of objects or weapons. Women and girls who suffer these injuries must cope with physical pain, leakage of urine and/or stool, psychological trauma, and the stigma and shame of the sexual assault itself.

Gender-based violence (GBV) resources and a skilled fistula surgical team are required to care for victims of sexual violence who develop a fistula. Patients often present malnourished with multiple other wounds, necessitating nutritional supplements to rebuild their strength and staged procedures to heal their wounds. Though some simple fistulas may be repaired during a single operation, complex fistulas often require multiple trips to the operating theater before a full reconstruction of all damaged organs is accomplished. The multidisciplinary mobilization of GBV therapies, advanced wound care, and staged surgical reconstruction must all be maintained for the duration of the fistula repair, which may take months to complete. For instance, most fistula care facilities lack general anesthetic capacity, so the fistula repairs are done with the patient awake under spinal anesthesia. The psychological trauma of repeated surgeries in lithotomy position after sexual violence cannot be understated. In fistula centers with limited sedation supplies, it is not uncommon for a GBV fistula patient to suffer flashbacks during each staged fistula operation.

Returning sexual violence fistula patients to their families, homes and communities presents strenuous challenges to fistula reintegration programs. Such reintegration must address the intricate mix of psychosocial traumas and stigma suffered by the patient and her family. Although the Nuremburg International Military Tribunal declared that rape was a crime against humanity, sexual violence continues to serve as a weapon of war. Despite this modern legal precedent, prosecuting cases of sexual violence during the 1998 Rwandan genocide trials proved difficult because of limited documentation of secondary injuries such as traumatic genital fistula. Since then, global stakeholder efforts to extensively document conflict zone sexual violence and resulting fistulas have increased. Detailed reports now exist from Angola, Burundi, Chad, Bosnia and Herzegovina, Chechnya, Democratic Republic of the Congo (DRC), Guinea, Haiti, India, Kosovo, Mozambique, Liberia, Pakistan, Peru, Serbia, Somalia, Uganda, Zimbabwe, and among displaced Somalis in Kenya, Burmese in Bangladesh, and Sudanese in Chad.

In 2005, the ACQUIRE project (Access, Quality, and Use in Reproductive Health) documented brutal rapes from Burundi, DRC, Liberia, Rwanda, Sierra Leone, and Sudan. In these accounts, thousands of women and girls, from the very young to the very old, were attacked. In addition to rape, the victims were subjected to other forms of physical and nonphysical abuse, including kidnapping and sexual slavery. Men and boys were also victims of sexual violence. The number of these sexually assaulted people who suffered genital fistulas, however, is not documented.

At a groundbreaking conference of the Ethiopian Society of Obstetricians and Gynecologists and Synergie des Femmes pour les Victimes des Violences Sexuelles held at the Addis Ababa Fistula Hospital in 2006, participants defined a list of factors known or believed to accelerate the risk and consequences of rape and the possibility of developing a genital fistula. These factors include armed conflict, internal and external displacement, community acceptance of gender-based and domestic violence, child marriage, child rape as a perceived method of HIV-status reversal, and female circumcision. Fistula surgeons at this conference reported a higher prevalence of unfixable fistulas caused by sexual violence compared to defects from obstructed labor or iatrogenic causes. The need for temporary colostomy, complex combined urinary and colorectal tract repairs carried out over several months, repair of adjacent soft tissue and abdominal organ damage, and counseling for profound psychological damage were also higher in the sexual violence group.

Recent public awareness of genital fistulas due to sexual violence comes mostly from reports from the eastern DRC, where decades of armed conflict have led to a high incidence of GBV and secondary genital fistulas. These reports documented sexual violence in 0.8% to 35% of fistula cases, with hospitals closer to the conflict zones reporting higher proportions of sexual etiologies among fistula patients. In addition, sexual and gender-based violence is perpetrated not only by rebel forces, but, due to the "normalization" of GBV in the eastern DRC, increasingly also by government troops, police, and even neighbors and relatives. A review of cases in 2005 at the Doctors On Call for Service (DOCS) Hospital in Goma found that the majority of fistulas admitted were secondary to sexual violence.

The high profile given to GBV-related fistula cases has generated interesting manipulations by patients. Some DRC fistula patients have believed that free fistula care was available only if they reported rape as the cause of their fistula, eventually admitting that their fistulas were due to obstructed labor. These untruths illustrate the capacity for humanitarian relief to cause the exact type of corruption it seeks to abolish and highlights the complex skill set needed to run a fistula service in a conflict zone.

A 2009 subanalysis of the Demographic and Health Surveys (DHS) data from Malawi, Rwanda, and Uganda estimated that elimination of sexual violence would result in a 7% to 40% reduction in the total burden of urinary and fecal incontinence. A more recent cross-sectional survey of women living in the Goma Province of eastern DRC found that sexual violence related to armed conflict was more likely to be associated with genital fistula than sexual violence unrelated to conflict. These findings likely reflect the higher prevalence of mass rape, sexual enslavement, and genital insertion of foreign bodies and weapons during conflict sexual assaults. Reports from areas known for sexual violence also illustrate the vulnerability of babies and young children, who, when sexually assaulted, are far more likely to sustain extensive soft tissue damage, including fistula.

Reports from the Hamlin Fistula Center in Addis Ababa, Ethiopia, document sexual violence–related fistulas occurring either "within marriage" *or* "due to rape." This illustrates the persistent notion that rape cannot occur within marriage, a phenomenon that coexists with child marriage, child abuse, GBV, and female circumcision as noncriminalized traditional conditions under which many women and girls continue to live.

The teenage student who survived the rebel abuse was ultimately transported several hundred miles away to a specialized fistula center for evaluation and management after her abdominal wounds were repaired at a hospital close to her home. The transfer of fistula patients to specialized centers is often necessary, as local surgical teams typically lack the soft tissue reconstructive skills, perioperative management expertise, and bed capacity necessary to address GBV genital fistulas.

The student required multiple staged operations over a 14-month period to fully restore her fecal and urinary continence and to reconstruct her genital tract to normal anatomy and fertility. Her mother eventually joined her at the fistula center. Funding was obtained to secure housing, food, and tuition so that they could live together near the center while awaiting the multiple reconstructive surgeries.

Despite the physical and psychological recuperation, like many victims of sexual violence, she continued to suffer from severe anxiety, panic attacks, attention deficits, flashbacks, and nightmares. Chronic pelvic pain and a morbid fear of sexual activity rendered her incapable of considering marriage. She was fortunate to have the support of her mother and to have found transport to a fistula center. She continues her studies at a university near the fistula hospital and plans to become a lawyer.

The global effort to reduce sexual violence is intrinsically related to the protection of human rights and evolving instruments of legal recourse. Public outcry and Western norms of sexual sovereignty as a human rights issue continue to conflict with local traditions and GBV perspectives. The challenge of preventing and treating genital fistula due to sexual violence mandates a coordinated effort. In addition to surgical capacity and skilled healthcare personnel, GBV genital fistula care highlights the necessity of psychosocial support, enforceable legislation, commensurate punishment of perpetrators, public awareness of the sexual aspects of human rights, timely access to sexual infection and pregnancy prevention and treatment, safe havens, and the paradoxical necessity of patience in the face of intolerable injustices.

Lauri J. Romanzi, MD, FACOG, FPMRS, is an urogynecologist with extensive humanitarian experience. Edna Adan Ismail, SRN, CMB, SCM, is a UK-trained nurse-midwife and was the first qualified nurse-midwife in Somaliland. She served as the WHO Representative in the Republic of Djibouti and as Minister of Social Affairs and Foreign Minister of Somaliland. In 2002 she founded the Edna Adan Maternity Hospital in Somaliland, and in 2012 opened the Edna Adan University.

ADDITIONAL READING

ACQUIRE Project. 2005. Traumatic gynecologic fistula as a consequence of sexual violence in conflict settings: a literature review. New York: The ACQUIRE Project / EngenderHealth. http://www.fistulacare.org/pages/pdf/traumatic_fistula_review—final.pdf (accessed March 5, 2016).

Addis Ababa Fistula Hospital, EngenderHealth / The ACQUIRE Project, Ethiopian Society of Obstetricians and Gynecologists, and Synergie des Femmes pour les Victimes des Violences Sexuelles. 2006. Traumatic gynecologic fistula: a consequence of sexual violence in conflict settings. New York: EngenderHealth/The ACQUIRE Project. http://www.engenderhealth.org/files/pubs/maternal-health/tf-report-english.pdf (accessed March 5, 2016).

Dossa NI, Zunzunegui MV, Hatem M, Fraser W. Fistula and other adverse reproductive health outcomes among women victims of conflict-related sexual violence: a population-based cross-sectional study. *Birth*. 2014 Mar;41(1):5–13. doi: 10.1111/birt.12085. PubMed PMID: 24654632.

Friends of UNFPA fact sheet on traumatic fistula. http://www.friendsofunfpa.org/netcommunity/page.aspx?pid=293 (accessed March 5, 2016).

Lancet Series: Violence against women and girls. http://www.thelancet.com/series/violence-against-women-and-girls (accessed March 5, 2016).

Obote-Odora, A. Rape and sexual violence in international law: ICTR contribution. *New Eng. J. Int'l & Comp. L.* 12, no. 1 ; 135–59.

Onsrud M, Sjøveian S, Luhiriri R, Mukwege D. Sexual violence–related fistulas in the Democratic Republic of Congo. *Int J Gynaecol Obstet.* 2008 Dec;103(3):265–9.

Peterman A, Johnson K. Incontinence and trauma: sexual violence, female genital cutting and proxy measures of gynecological fistula. *Soc Sci Med.* 2009 Mar;68(5):971–9.

World Health Organization. World report on violence and health. Chapter 6: Sexual violence. http://www.who.int/violence_injury_prevention/violence/world_report/en/ (accessed March 5, 2016).

World Health Organization. 2014 Global status report on violence prevention. http://www.who.int/violence_injury_prevention/violence/status_report/en/ (accessed March 5, 2016).

III   A WAY FORWARD

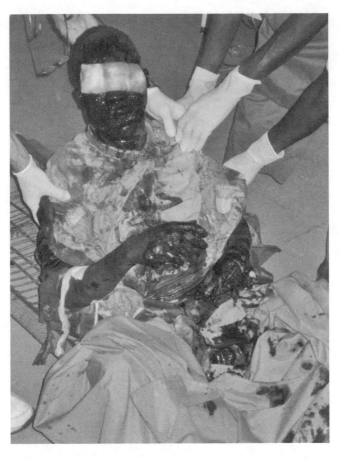

11.1. Land mine victim in South Sudan. Photo courtesy Adam L. Kushner

Advocating for a Cause

Documenting Land Mine Injuries in Cambodia

JAMES C. COBEY, MD, MPH, FACS

Land mines are considered "a weapon of mass destruction in slow motion." In 1991, the nongovernmental organization (NGO) Human Rights Watch (HRW) sought the assistance of Physicians for Human Rights (PHR) to document the problem of land mines in Cambodia. Prior to this, there were limited epidemiological data on the damage caused by these weapons to a civilian population after conflict. Since anecdotal evidence existed in Cambodia about a massive land mine problem affecting the population, HRW and PHR chose this Southeast Asian country for an initial study.

PHR, founded in 1986, differs from other human rights and advocacy groups, such as HRW and Amnesty International, by using scientific methods to collect data and describe the nature and size of human rights issues. To document the burden of land mines, two public health techniques could have been used, surveillance or surveys. Surveillance involves continually collecting data. The problem with surveillance is that data collection can take months or even years. In addition, data quality is highly dependent on individual data collectors. From personal experience of the author, surveys with motivated staff can be completed quickly and repeated months or years later for comparison. As the number of injuries from land mines was thought to be increasing, there was a need to act quickly, and so a survey approach was selected.

There are two main methods to collect data for land mine injury surveys, health facility–based reviews of medical records or community-based household interviews. The PHR/HRW study in Cambodia assessed hospital records, since it was easier to organize and quicker to implement. One problem with a hospital-based survey is that it will miss victims who never go to a medical facility because an injury is too small or the person died before receiving medical assistance. A community survey may be able to document these missing data but takes more time and resources. In addition, household members may or may not remember specifics about when and how a family member was wounded or died.

Historically, the concept of buried or underground explosives has existed since at least 1683, when the Turks dug tunnels under Vienna and planted explosives to destroy important structures. Land mines, as opposed to sea mines for targeting ships, became popular at the end of World War I to stop tanks. Initially, smaller land mines were used to protect the larger land mines from easily being removed. In World War II, both the Germans and British spread land mines throughout North Africa. Egypt still remains the most heavily infested country in the world, with an estimated 40 million unexploded land mines.

Small land mines are mostly deployed for defensive purposes. However, during the Vietnam War, many land mines planted by the United States were moved by the Vietnamese and caused a large number of the war injuries suffered by US soldiers. Researchers have also documented incidents where armies planted land mines in one area and then marched back through the same area a few months later with subsequent injuries to their own troops. After hostilities, armies often do not remove land mines because of the time, resources, or risks associated with removal. In many locations, maps of land mine–infested areas are poorly drawn or nonexistent. When not removed after a conflict, land mines pollute the land indefinitely, because the explosives can be active for many decades. In the United States, unexploded artillery shells from the 1860s Civil War are still occasionally found and can be lethal if set off.

When classifying land mines, there are two basic types: antitank and antipersonnel. Antitank land mines are large (10–20 kg explosives) and need a heavy pressure or force, usually from a vehicle, to cause a detonation. In addition, large land mines can be booby-trapped and set off when tampered with. Antipersonnel land mines are smaller (0.25–1 kg explosives) and designed primarily to wound rather than kill, since a wounded soldier requires more resources in terms of transport and assistance than a dead one.

Land mines can cause injury either directly from the blast effect of the explosive charge or by fragments that are propelled into the victim. General activation methods and categories of land mines include pressure, trip wire, bounding, scatterable, and unexploded "submunitions," or cluster bombs. Pressure mines are cheap to produce ($1–$20) and easy to deploy. They are detonated by only a few pounds of pressure, usually from being stepped on. Trip wire land mines are detonated when a victim disrupts a thin wire placed across a path; often, these are fragmentation land mines. Bounding land mines contain two charges. When activated, a small charge propels the main explosive a meter into the air. A second charge then propels fragments up to 30 meters. These land mines often kill the victim that caused the detonation and wound others who are nearby.

Scatterable land mines are deployed by artillery shells or dropped from helicopters. They are small, often look like toys, and injure victims by blast. Cluster bombs are containers of upward of 200 submunitions, each slightly larger than antipersonnel land mines. They can be launched by artillery or dropped from helicopters or planes. Though most cluster munitions detonate in the air or on impact, around 30% do not. These unexploded submunitions become de facto land mines with a much higher killing force than simple antipersonnel land mines. The mortality rate from a land mine injury is over 40% and from a submunition is over 70%.

The International Committee of the Red Cross (ICRC) classifies land mine injuries based on the pattern of injury. For the ICRC system:

Type I: The most common type (more than 60%) is an injury from stepping on a pressure-sensitive land mine. The blast destroys one foot and leg and severely injures the other side. With these injuries, soil, footwear and clothing, and fragments of bone are propelled up into the victim's leg and magnify the damage.

Type II: An injury from setting off a trip wire or bounding land mine. Fragments cause injuries to the abdomen or chest as well as legs.

Type III: An injury from picking up or trying to deactivate a land mine. The blast or fragments injure fingers, hands, and face, and often cause blindness. These injuries are most commonly seen in curious children or soldiers attempting to remove a land mine.

Most land mine injuries are severe. If the victim survives he or she will need to be treated in a hospital. In land mine–affected regions in many low-

and middle-income countries (LMICs), the ICRC or other NGOs run facilities with appropriate expertise and provide care for free. Local government facilities are frequently less well equipped. Also, while government hospitals may have the staff and beds, they often lack sufficient supplies. Frequently, family members must pay for services and provide medications, disposable supplies, and donors for blood transfusions. Postoperative nursing is also limited; therefore, family members often provide the basic care.

Many land mine injuries lead to amputation. An effective prosthesis can restore mobility and limit disability after a below-knee amputation. Above-knee and arm prostheses are more difficult to fit and victims, especially in LMICs, rarely get full function back. In some LMICs, an excellent below-knee prosthesis can be made locally for under $50. International organizations such as the ICRC, Handicap International, and others make prostheses and establish rehabilitation centers. However, they use imported components and they eventually leave. Victims will continually need care, and prosthetics wear out and will need replacements. Therefore, local solutions with locally procured components, locally assembled, and distributed by local personnel are best.

For the land mine injury survey in Cambodia, PHR assembled a three-person team that included a British land mine expert, a US human rights advocate and writer, and the author, a US orthopedic surgeon with a background in epidemiology. The goal was to estimate the burden of land mine injuries and document any issues.

The plan for the Cambodia study was to collect data from hospitals, but the question remained: how best to accomplish this? In LMICs, hospital surgical data can be difficult to access, especially when there is no standardized coding system. Looking through medical records is difficult, as individual physicians often record injuries differently. Fortunately, most operating rooms in LMICs have logbooks where all procedures are recorded. The survey team visited hospitals and recorded data on procedures performed for land mine victims. The procedures included mostly debridements and amputations. The logbook entries were written in legible French. As is well documented by the ICRC and other humanitarian organizations, for land mine injuries, many patients had two or three surgical procedures, so care was needed not to count victims twice. Analysis of the data estimated that

36,000 land mine victims existed in a population of 8.6 million. This meant that in Cambodia, 1 out of every 236 persons was a land mine victim.

Traveling around the country was difficult for the survey team because of the destroyed roads and limited infrastructure. In addition to the quantitative data from the logbooks, interviews with land mine victims provided qualitative information on the types of injuries and testimonies of the experience. Personal recollections included:

- If you step on a mine, you hope someone heard it and may come to your aid.
- Often people are afraid to help you by walking across a minefield.
- Many rescuers have died from mine injuries by trying to help a victim.
- Sometimes you have to cut your own leg off to be able to drag yourself to the side of the road and get help.

In Cambodia, help meant at least two people carrying the victim in a sling made from a blanket and a pole, and walking for miles to find someone with an oxcart or possibly a motor vehicle for transport to a hospital. The survey team also found that families kept a stack of land mines inside their homes. At night they would place them around their rice paddies for protection. In the morning, children would bring the land mines back inside. In the process, many land mines would accidentally detonate and result in blindness or the loss of fingers and hands.

When the survey team came back from Cambodia, efforts were made to disseminate the data and begin formal efforts to ban the weapon. HRW published a book, *Land Mines in Cambodia: The Coward's War,* which was distributed in the United States to the White House, Departments of Defense and State, all senators and members of Congress, and United Nations staffers. Initially, when the ICRC was asked to collect and publish their land mine injury data they refused, claiming it would compromise their neutrality.

Internationally, weapons data were historically handled under the Hague Treaty of 1898. Ultimately, the ICRC began to collect data at its own health facilities using forms similar to the ones developed by the PHR/HRW team. After a few months of data collection, the ICRC acknowledged the enormous burden of land mine injuries and considered it a major public health problem as well. Based on the initial data, it was estimated that one person was killed or injured by a land mine every 22 minutes. What also makes land mines even more horrific is that most victims are civilians, either women or children, living in areas where conflict has ceased long ago.

To raise awareness and work to end the use of land mines, PHR and HRW, along with Handicap International, Vietnam Veterans Association of America, Mines Advisory Group, and Medico International joined together and formed the International Campaign to Ban Landmines (ICBL). Jody Williams, an activist, was appointed as campaign coordinator. ICBL members began contacting other NGOs and professional organizations in an effort to get them to join the effort to stop the use of land mines. Currently, organizations from over 100 countries are members of the ICBL.

The initial ICBL work began with HRW staffers attempting to modify and extend the international treaty, the Convention on Conventional Weapons. Later, at a meeting in Geneva in 1993, government representatives debated the issue, but no firm plan was created. The US government initially supported the process but asked that weapons designed to self-destruct or stop working still be allowed. At this initial meeting in Geneva, NGOs were only allowed as observers and not allowed to speak. ICRC, which is recognized as an international organization, spoke as an expert on international humanitarian law.

No significant progress was made until October 1996, when the Canadian government offered to host a meeting for countries wishing to ban land mines. That meeting changed the course of how arms control negotiations are carried out. NGOs were allowed to participate and spoke directly with government representatives. At the meeting, it was agreed that the participants would move to draft a treaty against the use of land mines and meet again in the fall of 1997.

The HRW staff and others worked with many small and medium-size countries to draft a treaty on banning the use, production, stockpiling, and transfer of land mines, and for their destruction. Most previous international arms control treaties took many years to draft. For example, the treaties on the prohibition of chemical weapons, biological weapons, and nuclear weapons took, on average, 26 years to draft and become international law.

In less than one year, civil society groups working with small and medium-size countries such as Austria, Belgium, Canada, Norway, and Mozambique, and without the major powers such as the United States, the United Kingdom, Russia, or China, had drafted a treaty. Despite not signing the treaty, the US Department of State staff was very helpful in explaining the process. A consensus treaty was finalized and signed in December 1997.

Because of the efforts taken to help create the Mine Ban Treaty, in 1997, Jody Williams and the ICBL were awarded the Nobel Peace Prize. To date, 161 countries have joined the Mine Ban Treaty, also known as the Ottawa Treaty. In the Western Hemisphere, only Cuba and the United States have not joined. The United States is also the only NATO member that has not joined. Thirty-five nations that have not joined include China, Israel, Iran, India, North Korea, Pakistan, Russia, and Saudi Arabia.

Although use of land mines has decreased dramatically since 1991, there are still millions buried in more than 50 countries around the world. Land mines destroy lives and families. Until there is universal agreement and commitment never to use these weapons again, innocent people will continue to be injured.

James C. Cobey, MD, MPH, FACS, is an orthopedic surgeon. In 1991 he was part of the PHR/HRW team that assessed land mine injuries in Cambodia. In 1997 he shared in the Nobel Peace Prize for the International Campaign to Ban Landmines.

ADDITIONAL READING

Cameron M, et al. *To walk without fear: the global movement to ban land mines.* Oxford University Press, Toronto, 1998.

Cobey J. Medical complications of antipersonnel land mines. *Bulletin of the American College of Surgeons.* American College of Surgeons, Chicago, 1996.

Human Rights Watch. *Land mines in Cambodia: the coward's war.* 1991.

International Committee of the Red Cross. *The worldwide epidemic of land mine injuries.* Geneva, 1995.

Physicians for Human Rights. *Measuring land mine incidents and injuries and the capacity to provide care.* PHR, Boston, 2000.

Sigal L. *Negotiating minefields: the land mine ban in American politics.* Routledge, New York, 2006.

Stover E, McGrath R, Cobey J. *Land mines in Cambodia: the coward's war.* Asia Watch, Washington, 1991.

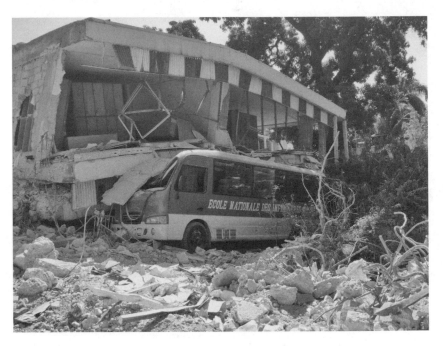
12.1. School of Nursing in Port au Prince, Haiti, after the Earthquake. Photo courtesy Dan L. Deckelbaum

12

Professionalizing Surgical Care in

Conflict and Disaster

The Haiti Earthquake and Beyond

EVAN G. WONG, MD, MPH, AND

DAN L. DECKELBAUM, MD, MPH, FACS

At 4:53 p.m., on January 12, 2010, a 7.0-magnitude earthquake struck Haiti. The epicenter was Léogâne, approximately 25 km west of Port-au-Prince, the capital. Over the next few days, aftershocks continued to rock the area. The consequences were devastating. Although estimates vary, the earthquake directly affected nearly 3 million people, 30% of the Haitian population. Over 250,000 homes were destroyed and 2.3 million persons displaced. An estimated 225,750 people died, and over 300,000 were injured, many needing surgical care.

The health system, limited at baseline, was quickly overwhelmed. In the days following the earthquake, multiple reports described extensive destruction of the existing healthcare infrastructure. The global community responded in force. The international humanitarian response was described among the largest nonconflict surgical responses in human history. Within three weeks of the quake, over 400 humanitarian organizations arrived in Haiti to assist with relief efforts. For many volunteers, this was their first experience with disaster relief. The response size led to much criticism, especially concerning surgical care. One positive effect was the recognition that more needed to be done to regulate and oversee international relief efforts.

Natural disasters, like most mass casualty incidents, disproportionately affect low-income countries. The surge in patients seeking care quickly consumes the limited resources. While injured persons seek care at nearby health facilities, these facilities are often also affected by the widespread destruction. In Haiti, approximately 60% of hospitals in the immediate vicinity of the epicenter were either severely damaged or completely destroyed. Many healthcare workers also died. As roads were blocked by rubble, basic necessities such as food, fuel, and shelter were unavailable.

Injured persons in Port-au-Prince saw that healthcare services were incapacitated. Anyone needing surgical care with access to a car, truck, or bus was immediately brought to one of the peripheral centers, in Deschapelles and Cange in Haiti, or Jimaní in the Dominican Republic. Also with limited capacity at baseline, these facilities were overwhelmed and within days resources were depleted. While barely publicized by the media nor documented in the medical literature, these peripheral centers, manned by local healthcare workers, played an essential role in providing emergency surgical care. While external organizations were mobilizing resources, local healthcare workers provided the life-saving care in those first hours and days. It is during this time that victims with potentially salvageable conditions die without access to care.

Reports on surgical care in the aftermath of earthquakes estimate that traumatic injuries, especially orthopedic trauma, predominate. As in conflict and other disaster settings, victims with significant head, chest, or abdominal injuries are unlikely to survive transport to the hospital. For patients with salvageable injuries to reach surgical care in time, it is imperative to minimize delays in supplying material and mobilizing resources.

A review of operations by international organizations immediately after the earthquake showed a predominance of amputations, wound debridements, and open fracture fixations. Delays in mobilizing more sophisticated surgical resources, however, probably resulted in much preventable death and disability.

The operative logbooks from a Canadian Forces field hospital set up 17 days after the earthquake noted mostly operations for chronic conditions, with only 13% for earthquake-related injuries. The most common procedures included hernia and hydrocele repairs, and hysterectomies. It is not uncommon that surgical responders to a disaster will encounter traumatic injuries and also routine acute and chronic surgical conditions.

Though triage is a hallmark of any conflict or disaster situation, the large number of Foreign Medical Teams (FMTs) and the importation of massive amounts of equipment and supplies created complex ethical dilemmas. Inexperienced volunteers encountered decisions that were beyond the scope of their routine practice. The Israeli Defense Forces described the ethical dilemmas encountered in their field hospital in a comment to the *New England Journal of Medicine*. They noted that patients were selected based on the urgency of their injuries, the availability of required resources, and the reversibility of their illnesses. Crush injuries, head trauma, and spinal injuries were examples of urgent conditions requiring extensive resources that might not be reversible. Extensive media coverage of patients saved after surviving days under rubble also created dilemmas. With so many nonmedical resources dedicated to the rescue, was refusing surgical care based on the underlying injuries ethical?

To deal with these difficult decisions, the Israelis created an ad hoc ethics committee to alleviate decision making from medical personnel in these situations. The committee comprised three senior physicians, who, after hearing the case from the treating physician, would deliberate and agree on a course of action. All decisions were then recorded in the patients' charts. The system distilled actionable instructions from complex situations and alleviated individual physicians from the burden of making life-and-death decisions based on limited resources. They recommended development of a preexisting ethical framework to be implemented prior to any disaster deployment.

Without preexisting disaster plans, health systems plummet into chaos after a natural disaster. In a low-resource setting such as Haiti, this led to even bigger problems. The involvement of external organizations and the influx of FMTs, without overarching supervision, compounded the difficulties. The response was inefficient. There was duplication of efforts and a disorganized distribution of resources. There was no supervision or certification, and limited accountability or quality control.

Although well meaning, which is typical but not always helpful, the massive influx of FMTs highlighted a number of issues. Multiple field hospitals deployed with little communication or coordination. The United Nations Office of the Coordination of Humanitarian Affairs (OCHA), the main coordinating body of the humanitarian response community, quickly established the Cluster Coordination System; yet, many of the FMTs were unfamiliar with this. With no criteria to be an FMT, surgical capabilities and quality varied greatly. Without an overall supervising body or established minimum standards of care, questionable clinical decisions were made. For example, a significant number of amputations were done, and reports document that many were unnecessary.

These problems with FMTs and the overall humanitarian response led to calls for professionalization and better coordination. In the aftermath of the response, Médecins Sans Frontières (MSF) reviewed its experience delivering surgical care and recommended increased effectiveness for surgical care disaster response. One key requirement is a supply of appropriate material and skilled personnel within the opportune window of time. This can be achieved through the preparation of emergency kits held in warehouses close to high-risk locations; preapproved importation agreements for medical supplies; and the ongoing training of surgical personnel specifically for humanitarian settings.

To professionalize response teams, the United Kingdom International Emergency Trauma Register, a formal inventory of surgeons, anesthesiologists, emergency physicians, nurses, and other auxiliary medical personnel who would be willing to help in the event of an emergency, was developed. This register has been revolutionary for several reasons. It permits a governing body to verify participants' credentials and skill set prior to deployment, thus ensuring a minimum level of training. Furthermore, by identifying individuals with different skill sets, the register promotes the formation of complementary teams and ensures that the right medical personnel are able to fulfill the medical needs of the specific emergency. A central register of deployable FMTs will improve coordination abroad and help identify replacements for deployed personnel at their home institutions. Finally, documentation of deployed FMTs will enhance accountability.

The World Health Organization recently developed minimal standards for FMTs in the event of a sudden onset disaster. Specifically for surgery, there are also now best practice guidelines for emergency care in disaster situations. These guidelines focus on key surgical concepts relevant to disasters, and particularly earthquakes, and include disinfection and sterilization, resuscitation, laceration repairs, amputations, fracture repairs, and the management of compartment syndrome and fat embolism syndrome. These standards can provide a means of certification to standardize care.

Surgical care in the aftermath of an earthquake presents a number of organizational challenges. The clinical response must rely on principles common to other natural disasters and mass casualty incidents, such as the oil pipeline explosion in Freetown, Sierra Leone, described in Chapter 5. The prompt mobilization of resources and the use of peripheral treatment centers are both critical for an efficient response. Ethical standards must be maintained, both in the triage of patients and in the quality of FMTs. Adequate coordination and communication between local and international teams is essential. Finally, working with local healthcare workers is fundamental; only through long-term collaboration and advances in baseline capacity will resilience of these communities improve.

Dan L. Deckelbaum, MD, MPH, FACS, is a trauma surgeon based at McGill University in Montreal, Canada. He arrived two days after the Haiti earthquake.

ADDITIONAL READING

Best practice guidelines on emergency surgical care in disaster situations. Geneva, Switzerland, World Health Organization, 2005.

Carlson LC, Hirshon JM, Calvello EJ, et al. Operative care after the Haiti 2010 earthquake: implications for post-disaster definitive care. *American Journal of Emergency Medicine* 2013: 31; 429–431.

Chu K, Stokes C, Trelles M, et al. Improving effective surgical delivery in humanitarian disasters: lessons from Haiti. *PLoS medicine* 2011: 8; e1001025.

Classification and minimum standards for foreign medical teams in sudden onset disasters. Geneva, Switzerland, World Health Organization, 2013.

Deckelbaum DL. The Haiti earthquake: a personal perspective. *CMAJ* 2010: 182; E241–242.

Kirsch T, Sauer L, Guha Sapir D. Analysis of the international and US response to the Haiti earthquake: recommendations for change. *Disaster Medicine and Public Health Preparedness* 2012: 6; 200–208.

McIntyre T, Hughes CD, Pauyo T, et al. Emergency surgical care delivery in post-earthquake Haiti: Partners in Health and Zanmi Lasante experience. *World Journal of Surgery* 2011: 35; 745–750.

Merin O, Ash N, Levy G, et al. The Israeli field hospital in Haiti—ethical dilemmas in early disaster response. *New England Journal of Medicine* 2010: 362; e38.

Redmond AD, O'Dempsey TJ, Taithe B. Disasters and a register for foreign medical teams. *Lancet* 2011: 377; 1054–1055.

Sullivan SR, Taylor HO, Pauyo T, et al. Surgeons' dispatch from Cange, Haiti. *New England Journal of Medicine* 2010: 362; e19.

Talbot M, Meunier B, Trottier V, et al. 1 Canadian Field Hospital in Haiti: surgical experience in earthquake relief. *Canadian Journal of Surgery* 2012: 55; 271–274.

Wong EG, Trelles M, Dominguez L, et al. Surgical skills needed for humanitarian missions in resource-limited settings: common operative procedures performed at Médecins Sans Frontières facilities. *Surgery* 2014 Sep;156(3):642–649.

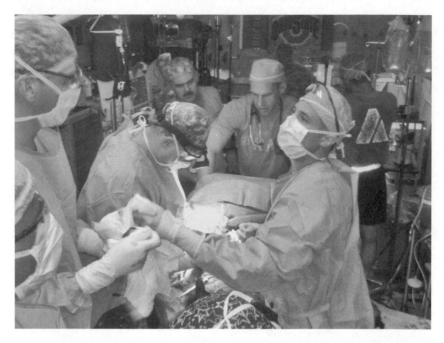
13.1. Operating at a Role 2 Forward Surgical Team in Afghanistan. Photo courtesy Kyle N. Remick

US Military Joint Trauma System and Roles of Care

LTC KYLE N. REMICK, MD, FACS,

AND COL JEFFREY A. BAILEY, MD, FACS

An improvised explosive device—the most common weapon used against US forces in Iraq and Afghanistan—detonated near a squad patrolling on foot in a small dusty village. One soldier was severely wounded. The explosive blast tore apart his legs; both were traumatically amputated. A cry of "MEDIC!!" went out and despite a hail of incoming small arms fire, a combat medic immediately rushed to the soldier's side and placed tourniquets on the bleeding stumps. This procedure saved a life but was just the first step of the US military Joint Trauma System (JTS).

The JTS is a military trauma system developed to care for battlefield injuries of US service members (soldiers, sailors, airmen, or marines). Despite the difficult and dangerous environment, it comprehensively includes transport, stabilization, definitive care, and rehabilitation. The journey from combat injury to rehabilitation and social reintegration takes from days to years. The system is designed to provide a stepped management of care along the way.

To optimally care for combat injuries, an organized system and well-trained staff are required. The North Atlantic Treaty Organization (NATO) defines standardized "Roles of Care" for military medicine. Role 1 is at the point of injury and encompasses the care provided by a combat medic. Role 2 is a forward facility near the front lines of fighting with a trauma team led by a physician or physician's assistant to provide initial resuscitation and possibly limited surgical care. Role 3 is typically a fixed-position hospital and is the last stop for a casualty within the theater of operations. Role 4 is definitive care outside the combat zone. For US casualties, Role 4 includes

Table 13.1. Roles of care definitions

Role 1	First aid, immediate lifesaving measures, and triage.
Role 2	Triage and resuscitation, treatment and holding of patients until returned to duty or evacuated, and emergency dental treatment. May augment with emergency surgery and essential postoperative management.
Role 3	Specialist diagnostic resources, specialist surgical and medical capabilities, preventive medicine, food inspection, dentistry, and operational stress management teams. Holding capacity to allow diagnosis, treatment, and holding of patients to receive total treatment and be returned to duty.
Role 4	Definitive care of patients for whom the treatment required is longer than the theater evacuation policy or for whom the capabilities at Role 3 are inadequate. Comprise specialist surgical and medical procedures, reconstruction, rehabilitation, and convalescence.
Role 5	Care provided in the Continental United States.

Landstuhl Regional Medical Center in Germany and subsequent care and rehabilitation provided by US military trauma centers in the United States.

When a US service member is wounded, a specially trained combat medic arrives at the point of injury within minutes. These medics undergo Tactical Combat Casualty Care training and learn to correct preventable causes of death on the battlefield. In general terms this means controlling compressible bleeding with a tourniquet; performing a cricothyroidotomy (placing a small breathing tube through the neck) for severe facial or neck trauma; and needle decompression of a tension pneumothorax (releasing pressure from a lung injury that can compress large blood vessels in the chest and lead to death). The training guidelines were developed for the realities of providing care during combat and are divided into three phases: Care under fire, Tactical field care, and Care during evacuation.

For the "Care under fire" phase, the medic uses tourniquets to stop life-threatening bleeding and then returns to the firefight. After the immediate fighting ceases, the "Tactical field care" phase involves moving the casualty to a safe location and performing a sequenced evaluation. Checks are performed for sources of catastrophic bleeding, for breathing, and to measure the pulse. The pulse and the casualty's level of alertness are used to assess the extent of blood loss. Critical injuries with greater blood loss will need quicker transport to the next role of care. An intravenous (in the vein) or intraosseous (in the bone) catheter is placed; however, fluids are only given for a worsening blood pressure as measured by decreased alertness.

The medic also radios the unit's tactical operations center at the forward operating base to request air medical evacuation (medevac). The US Army "Huey" and "Blackhawk" helicopters, commonly known by the call sign "Dust-off," have played a key role in the evacuation of battlefield casualties for over 50 years. The 57th Medical Detachment (Air Ambulance) first used this call sign in Vietnam in 1963, when pilots made their reputation by flying through hailstorms of bullets to collect the wounded. This call sign has since become synonymous with helicopter evacuation from the battlefield.

In the helicopter, specially trained flight medics care for the casualty from the evacuation site to the next role of care and provide "Care during evacuation." Despite the noisy, vibrating, and limited space to maneuver in the helicopter, flight medics reassess the level of consciousness to check for massive blood loss and dangerously low blood pressure. Blood for transfusion is onboard and key to survival for some casualties. Additionally, the medevac helicopter carries equipment such as pelvic binders to slow internal bleeding from a pelvic fracture. The medevac flights are short, sometimes as quick as 5 to 10 minutes. Casualties typically are taken directly to a secure base with a Role 2 surgical capability such as an Army Forward Surgical Team. The time from injury in a remote location to the Role 2 facility with surgical capabilities is, in many cases, less than 30 minutes.

A physician, basic laboratory and radiologic capability, and capacity to keep a casualty for a period of time are the hallmarks of a Role 2 facility. The US military predominantly uses Role 2 locations as the first site for surgical care and designates them as "Role 2—Surgical." These facilities are located near the front lines. Resource and personnel are relatively limited. The surgical team, consisting of surgeons, anesthesia providers, nurses, and enlisted medical personnel focus on one mission—combat trauma care. They operate in tents or in plywood or cement buildings. Usually, the facilities are not as clean as would be expected in a US hospital. Facilities can also be easily overwhelmed when more than four casualties arrive simultaneously or more than two require immediate surgery.

A key concept in the initial management of a severely injured casualty is damage control resuscitation, rapidly providing blood and blood products to prevent or reverse the trauma triad of death: hypothermia (low temperature), coagulopathy (poor clotting), and acidosis. Over the last decade, data have showed that providing a 1:1:1 ratio of red blood cells to plasma to platelets reduced mortality, especially in the most severely injured casualties. Most Role 2—Surgical facilities maintain a supply of red blood cells and plasma but not platelets. Consequently, casualties needing large-volume transfusions or platelets are transfused with fresh whole blood from pre-screened, primarily US volunteers on the base. This fresh whole blood contains all the necessary components in the appropriate ratio.

Role 2—Surgical teams are also trained to provide life-saving damage control surgery. While tourniquets prevent life-threatening bleeding from extremity injuries, bleeding in the chest, abdomen, and pelvis needs more definitive care. Combat surgeons can quickly identify and stop this torso bleeding and minimize contamination from injured intestines. The underlying principle of damage control surgery is to do everything needed to save life or limb, but nothing more. A Role 2—Surgical facility is not designed for delicate, technically challenging, or time-consuming procedures. If a team tries to do too much for one casualty, other injured service members who arrive afterward might not receive life- or limb-saving care. Examples of damage control surgery techniques include rapid removal of injured or leaking intestines; controlling heart, major chest, or abdominal blood vessels; and using plastic tubes to temporarily shunt arm or leg blood vessels for definitive repair at a later time. After a damage control procedure, a temporary abdominal closure is rapidly done with a towel, plastic cover, and suction to protect the abdominal contents.

For the blast injuries typically seen in combat, damage control techniques and multiple surgeons are needed. General/trauma surgeons will explore an abdomen or chest to stop bleeding and contamination. Orthopedic surgeons remove debris such as dirt, uniform material, and dead tissue from the wound and stabilize broken bones. The general surgeons also explore and remove debris and dead tissue from the perineum, the area around the scrotum and anus. The now widespread use of armored pelvic undergarments is an example of innovation and injury prevention, which has led to a decrease in the frequency and severity of these injuries.

After evaluation and stabilization at the Role 2, the wounded service member is transported to the Role 3 facility, which is usually considered a "theater hospital." Transport from Role 2 to Role 3 facilities and beyond often requires more advanced training and specialized skills. A team of an advanced flight medic and a critical care–trained flight nurse provides intensive in-flight care. Often, casualties undergo surgery at the Role 2 and are still sedated and intubated (chemically unconscious with a tube for breathing) for the journey to the Role 3 facility. They need special transport equipment and support.

A Role 3 facility is as close to a modern trauma hospital as possible within the combat zone. It has a larger capacity than the Role 2 facility, with increased capability and resources. A neurosurgeon and a CT scanner make the Role 3 the ideal location to treat head-injured casualties. Other subspecialists such as plastic surgeons and neck and face surgeons are usually available to perform complex facial reconstructions. There is an intensive care unit to provide ongoing in-theater casualty resuscitation and critical care. Despite the increased resources, Role 3 facilities do face personnel and resource limitations during periods of intense fighting or after mass casualty incidents. Although the Role 3 often looks and feels like a hospital in the United States, the enemy is still nearby and attack is possible.

Upon arrival at the Role 3 facility, the casualty is thoroughly reevaluated. More blood is available if needed, and a CT scan can help identify additional injuries. The temporary abdominal closures, initial amputations, and temporary shunts done to save life and limb at the Role 2 are reopened for examination and further surgery. After surgery, the casualty often requires continued intensive care prior to transport out of the theater of war.

The US Air Force Critical Care Air Transport Team, or CCATT, is specially trained to care for wounded service members on a fixed-wing aircraft for long flight times. The teams have refined their skills over the past decade and are able to care for the most severely injured combat casualties in a confined environment. They are also knowledgeable as to how altitude affects physiology in critically ill patients. As some flights can take 10 hours, the CCATT is essentially a flying intensive care unit "on an island" and must be self-sufficient, since there are no other specialists who can help should the casualty's status deteriorate.

The Role 4 facility for US service members wounded in Iraq or Afghanistan is Landstuhl Regional Medical Center in Germany. After a long CCATT transport, the trauma team in Landstuhl reevaluates all injuries once again. A true multispecialty trauma team reviews each casualty daily and more frequently if needed. This team includes trauma surgeons, critical care physicians, critical care nurses, nutritionists, physical therapists, respiratory therapists, and other subspecialty surgeons as needed. The trauma program managers and US Air Force transport specialists also coordinate and time the next long transport to a military trauma center in the United States.

Usually for a third time, the casualty's wounds are reevaluated and worked on in an operating room. The hospital and operating room, however, now offer a clean environment where operative sterility is on par with US hospitals. This begins the transition of damage control to definitive surgery. Reconstruction of extremities and the closure of complex wounds will still come later.

When ready for transport back to the United States, the CCATT again provides the essential critical care. Severely injured service members are transported to one of two main military trauma hospitals, San Antonio Military Medical Center in Texas or Walter Reed National Military Medical Center in Maryland. Although NATO designates these facilities as Role 4, since they are outside the theater of war, the US Military adds a Role 5 designation for US-based trauma centers.

At the Role 5 facility, a full spectrum of definitive trauma care is provided. Definitive abdominal and amputation wound closures are performed, and invasive tubes and lines are sequentially removed as the physiologic damage of the trauma resolves. The casualty regains consciousness and is reunited with family and loved ones. Over the course of weeks and months, wounds heal and care transitions to the rehabilitation phase of trauma care.

Behind the physical set-up of the roles of care for battlefield injuries is the JTS. This military trauma system was created in 2004 and modeled on the success of civilian trauma systems with modifications to account for combat. The vision was "to get the right patient to the right place at the right time."

A systems approach to combat trauma care facilitated improvements within each component area. Military trauma system leadership was established in the form of the theater trauma director, who was given direct access to the highest levels of operational leadership to allow data col-

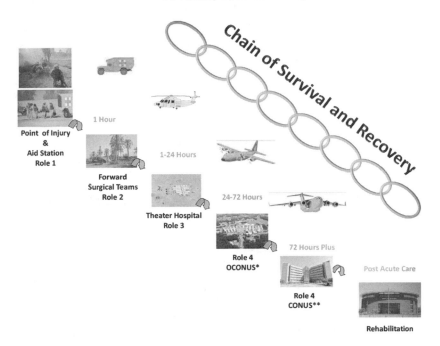

13.2. Joint Trauma System Continuum of Care, OCONUS = Outside Continental US; CONUS = Inside Continental US

lection, analysis, and rapid feedback regarding initiatives that could save lives. In the area of prevention, improved body armor decreased thoracic trauma from 18% to less than 5%. Increased armor on vehicles decreased the number and severity of vehicle blast injuries. In the area of battlefield care, mortal battlefield hemorrhage from extremity injury was decreased by the use of tourniquets and hemostatic dressings. In the realm of quality improvement, electronic medical records were established to facilitate communication between roles of care on the battlefield and with Landsthuhl in Germany and the medical centers in the United States. Furthermore, a trauma registry was established and data collection was initiated. Teams of registry personnel deployed to theaters of operations under the supervision of the Trauma Director to collect data and perform real-time analysis. This allowed for timely feedback to commanders, and it generated life-saving changes to the system. Lastly, important lessons were captured in the form of clinical guidelines to standardize practice across the trauma system continuum of care.

In essence, the JTS revolutionized battlefield trauma care. It now formally provides a trauma system that spans the globe from the point of injury on the battlefield through all of the roles of care described and to rehabilitation in the United States. The JTS has taken lessons learned from urban and civilian trauma systems and created a system in a combat context with global reach back to the United States. The strength of the system optimizes resources but also helps to save lives and reduce disabilities.

Disclaimer: The opinions presented are those of the authors only and do not necessarily represent the views of the US Army, Marines, Navy, or Air Force, the Department of Defense, or the US government.

ADDITIONAL READING

Bailey J, Spott MA, Costanzo GP, et al. *Joint trauma system: development, conceptual framework, and optimal elements*. US Department of Defense, US Army Institute for Surgical Research, 2012.

Beninati W, Meyer MT, Carter TE. The critical care air transport program. *Crit Care Med*. 2008; 36[Suppl.]:S370–S376.

Blackbourne LH. Combat damage control surgery. *Crit Care Med*. 2008; 36[Suppl.]: S304–S310.

Borgman MA, Spinella PC, Perkins JG, et al. The ratio of blood products transfused affects mortality in patients receiving massive transfusions at a combat support hospital. *J Trauma*. 2007;63:805–813.

Celso B, Tepas J, Langland-Orban B, et al. A systematic review and meta-analysis comparing outcome of severely injured patients treated in trauma centers following the establishment of trauma systems. *J Trauma*. 2006; 60:371–378.

Dorlac GR, Fang R, Pruitt VM, et al. Air transport of patients with severe lung injury: development and utilization of the acute lung rescue team. *J Trauma*. 2009;66:S164–S171.

Dorland P, and Nanney J. *Dust off: Army aeromedical evacuation in Vietnam*. US Government Printing Office, Washington, DC. 1982.

Duchesne JC, McSwain NE, Cotton BA, et al. Damage control resuscitation: the new face of damage control. *J Trauma*. 2010;69(4): 976–990.

Eastridge BJ, Jenkins D, Flaherty S, et al. Trauma system development in a theater of war: experiences from Operation Iraqi Freedom and Operation Enduring Freedom. *J Trauma*. 2006; 61:1366–1373.

Eastridge BJ, Mabry RL, Seguin P, et al. Death on the battlefield (2001–2011): implications for the future of combat casualty care. *J Trauma Acute Care Surg*. 2012;73:S431–S437. FM 4-02.2 Medical Evacuation. May 2007. Available at *http://armypubs.army.mil/doctrine* (accessed March 5, 2016).

Haas B, Jurkovich GJ, Wang J, et al. Survival advantage in trauma centers: expeditious intervention or experience? *J Am Coll Surg.* 2009; 208:28–36.

Kelly JF, Ritenour AE, McLaughlin DF, et al. Injury severity and causes of death from Operation Iraqi Freedom and Operation Enduring Freedom: 2003–2004 versus 2006. *J Trauma.* 2008;64:S21–S27.

Kotwal RS, Montgomery HR, Kotwal BM, et al. Eliminating preventable death on the battlefield. *Arch Surg.* 2011;146(12):1350–1358.

MacKenzie EJ, Rivara FP, Jurkovich GJ, et al. A national evaluation of the effect of trauma-center care on mortality. *N Engl J Med.* 2006; 354:366–378.

Nessen SC, Eastridge BJ, Cronk D, et al. Fresh whole blood use by forward surgical teams in Afghanistan is associated with improved survival compared to component therapy without platelets. *Transfusion.* 2013;53:107S–113S.

Perkins JG, Cap AP, Spinella PC, et al. Comparison of platelet transfusion as fresh whole blood versus apheresis platelets for massively transfused combat trauma patients. *Transfusion.* 2011;51:242–252.

West JG, Trunkey DD, Lim RC. Systems of trauma care, *Arch Surg.* 1979; 114:455–460.

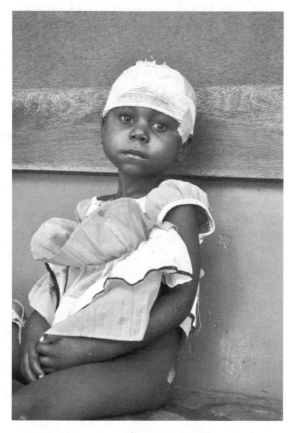

C.1. A victim of conflict in the Democratic Republic of the Congo. Photo courtesy Chiels Liu

Conclusion

BARCLAY T. STEWART, MD, MSCPH,

AND ADAM L. KUSHNER, MD, MPH, FACS

Dramatic images, videos, and media reports from modern crises now reach around the globe. Often, there seems little can be done to help the wounded during conflict or after a disaster. Certainly many victims will die, lose limbs, or become disabled. Yet despite the difficulties in rendering care, with proper training and planning much can be done to limit excess death, disability, and suffering.

In the developing world, preventable deaths and disabilities are routine occurrences because of baseline health system deficiencies. During conflict or disasters, most health systems deteriorate further, and so does the quality of care. Civilians, especially vulnerable populations such as women, children, and the elderly, bear the greatest burden of the collapse.

The chapters of this book included vignettes that highlight the challenges and successes of providing surgical care in a variety of crises. Each of these crises had unique features. However, the cases have demonstrated several central tenets that, when followed, ensure safe, effective, and responsible treatment: adhere to the principles of war surgery and wound management; have deference for local colleagues and existing healthcare systems; be committed to ethics and humanitarian principles; and adapt and innovate.

The contributors to this book have provided valuable insights and lessons learned from personal experiences of providing surgical and obstetric care in some of the most devastating crises of this generation. The stories highlight how working during conflict or disaster is taxing and requires an extraordinary breadth of skill and understanding of both personal and contextual limitations. In Part I, personal perspectives highlight the day-to-day work of general and orthopedic surgeons and obstetrician/ gynecologists. Despite all the obstacles, however, the authors have demonstrated that with a well-planned surgical response, satisfactory outcomes can be achieved, even in the most austere settings.

Understanding and following established surgical principles during conflict and disaster are key to saving lives, minimizing disabilities, and conserving limited resources. Failure to adhere to these principles can lead to unnecessary deaths and complications, longer hospital stays, unnecessary operations, and needless use of scarce supplies. Dr. Robin Coupland, former head of war surgery for the ICRC, put forth several important recommendations in his landmark paper, "Epidemiological Approach to Surgical Management of the Casualties of War." In the paper, he described lessons from his experience as a war surgeon:

1. Many patients, even with severe injuries, do not necessarily require surgery to survive for many days or even weeks.
2. Appropriate surgical skills and equipment are difficult to import and may not be usable under difficult or dangerous circumstances.
3. Inadequate surgery is worse than nothing.
4. A basic level of nursing care could achieve much.
5. Intravenous fluids and antibiotics buy time for most patients.
6. Patients with severe, life-threatening injuries die despite treatment unless resources, the number of nursing staff, and the organization of the hospital infrastructure are adequate.
7. When the hospital infrastructure is disrupted surgical resources are easily wasted by operating on patients whose prognosis is hopeless— underlining the importance of realistic triage for treatment—and the death rate is unacceptably high among those who should survive the surgery.

Dr. Coupland's conclusions were controversial, so much so that he received death threats when his paper was published. The observations he offered were from years of war surgery experience. These important lessons for providing surgical care appropriate for the circumstances are valid not only in war but also during disasters, and even in settings that lack sufficient infrastructure, trained healthcare personnel, or physical resources to provide advanced care.

Part II goes beyond the personal recounting of experiences and offers many of the more technical topics needed to provide surgical care: triage and training (Chapter 5), wound management (Chapter 6), burns (Chapter 7), anesthesia (Chapter 8), women's health (Chapter 9), and sexual violence (Chapter 10). Again, these chapters afford personal experience and lessons learned from those with on-the-ground experience.

An important caveat is that local healthcare workers and volunteers provide the majority of care during conflicts and disasters. Although most of the authors in this book worked with international organizations, it is important to recognize that their experiences are quite different from the healthcare professionals who provided care in their home environment during these difficult conditions, such as in Chapter 1. One aim of this book is to educate and inform volunteers who wish to work for humanitarian organizations such as ICRC or MSF. Unprepared personnel may have difficulty providing quality care due to the stress and unfamiliarity of these unrelentingly intense situations. International and national staff should work closely to share the skills required for meeting patients' needs and the knowledge required to practice surgical care with minimal resources.

In addition to principles of war surgical care, universal medical ethics with consideration of humanitarian principles should be followed. Tenets of patient autonomy, informed consent, confidentiality, beneficence, and nonmaleficence are easily forgotten during intensely stressful times, but universal adherence is a must. In addition, humanitarian medical teams should be versed in and practice the field's defining principles:

1. Humanity—all humankind should be treated humanely and their dignity upheld in all circumstances
2. Impartiality—assistance should not be based on nationality, race, religion, or political perspective but on need alone
3. Independence—aid is devised independent of government actions or policies
4. Neutrality—avoidance of choosing a side during conflict or engaging in controversies of political, religious, racial, or ideological nature when possible

By following these principles, healthcare workers can provide care to victims of crisis with respect and humanity. Also future humanitarian aid in complex political situations will not be jeopardized and the safety of staff and patients maintained to the best of a team's ability.

The authors also identified and discussed issues going beyond the operating room, such as precrisis surgical team registration and response planning, crisis medical team organization and overarching coordination, and long-term restoration of health and surgical systems within local healthcare contexts. As these precepts continue to become standards in the humanitarian surgical framework, the discipline of humanitarian surgery will continue to evolve into a practice of its own. The chapters on disasters in Sierra Leone (Chapter 5), Indonesia (Chapter 6), and Haiti (Chapter 12) taught us that all countries are at some risk of conflict or disaster and should consider these precepts to create their own national or local emergency response plans.

Having developed an understanding of the complexities surrounding healthcare delivery during conflict or disaster, surgical healthcare workers are in a unique position to advocate for greater standards of care; increased resources; better training; enhanced communication and coordination; and human rights of those affected by crisis. Part III looked at what could be done to move forward. Chapter 11 covered the use of data and effects of advocacy that led to the Mine Ban Treaty and a massive reduction in resulting antipersonnel land mine injuries. Chapter 12 addressed issues with the humanitarian response after the Haiti earthquake and the need to develop credentials for humanitarian responders. Chapter 13 described the US military Joint Trauma System and showed the type of care that can be rendered in difficult and dangerous situations if there are sufficient resources and political will.

The need for adaptability when working in low-resource settings should go without saying; however, eager but unskilled volunteers have been a hallmark of international relief operations. Anecdotal stories of staff arriving in Haiti after the 2010 earthquake demanding to be supplied with relatively costly resources and nonlocal food abound. To ensure that the spirit of volunteerism does not degenerate into "voluntourism," international organizations are improving the way staff are recruited, organized, and managed.

As described in Chapter 12, examples of professionalizing humanitarian care are evolving. Initiatives such as the United Kingdom International

Emergency Trauma Register, the United Nations cluster system, and the SPHERE project are but a few examples. Together, these initiatives identify and help deploy qualified staff who then work under predefined standards of care so that the humanitarian response occurs quickly, safely, and effectively. Continuing efforts to professionalize humanitarian surgical care are important and will certainly lead to better outcomes for victims of future crises.

Ultimately, it is hoped that by sharing these personal experiences of providing surgical care in conflict and disaster, this book offers inspiration, instruction, and insight into the extraordinary opportunity to deliver care for those most in need. As these examples demonstrate, being a part of a surgical team during crisis is a humbling but rewarding privilege. Most of all, providing surgical care during crisis has the potential to avert an extraordinary amount of death and disability.

ADDITIONAL READING

Bae JY, Groen RS, Kushner AL. Surgery as a public health intervention: common misconceptions versus the truth. *Bull World Health Organ.* 2011 Jun 1;89(6):394.

Chu KM, Ford N, Trelles M. Operative mortality in resource-limited settings: the experience of Médecins Sans Frontières in 13 countries. *Arch Surg.* 2010 Aug;145(8):721–5.

Coupland RM. Epidemiological approach to surgical management of the casualties of war. *BMJ.* 1994 Jun 25;308(6945):1693–7.

The Sphere Project. *Humanitarian charter and minimum standards in humanitarian response. http://www.sphereproject.org* (accessed March 4, 2016).

WHO. *International humanitarian norms and principles.* World Health Organization, Interagency Standing Committee, Geneva, Switzerland: 2010.

Index

Page numbers in *italics* indicate photographs.